T022454?

Antiquarianism, Language, and Medical Philology

Antiquarianism, Language, and Medical Philology

*From Early Modern to Modern Sino-Japanese
Medical Discourses*

Edited by

Benjamin A. Elman

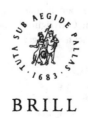

BRILL

LEIDEN | BOSTON

This paperback was originally published in hardback as Volume 12 in the Sir Henry Wellcome Asian Series.

Based on a "Research Cluster" supported by the Princeton Institute for International and Regional Studies and the East Asian Studies Program, 2009–2012. Thanks are also due the Davis Center for History and the Council for the Humanities Gardner Fund for their support. A Mellon Foundation Career Achievement Award provided a timely publication subvention for the project.

Cover illustration: The cut-and-paste version of Yang Shoujing's edition of the *Shanghan lun* (Treatise on Cold Damage Disorders) in the National Central Library, Taipei.

The Library of Congress Cataloging-in-Publication Data has catalogued the hardcover edition as follows:

Antiquarianism, language, and medical philology : from early modern to modern Sino-Japanese medical discourses / edited by Benjamin A. Elman.
p. ; cm. -- (Sir Henry Wellcome Asian series, ISSN 1570-1484 ; volume 12)
Includes bibliographical references and index.
ISBN 978-90-04-28544-6 (hardback : alk. paper) -- ISBN 978-90-04-28545-3 (e-book)
I. Elman, Benjamin A., 1946- , editor. II. Series: Sir Henry Wellcome Asian series (Brill Academic Publishers) ; v. 12. 1570-1484
[DNLM: 1. Medicine, East Asian Traditional--history--China. 2. Medicine, East Asian Traditional--history--Japan. 3. History, 18th Century--China. 4. History, 18th Century--Japan. 5. History, Ancient--China. 6. History, Ancient--Japan. 7. History, Early Modern 1451-1600--China. 8. History, Early Modern 1451-1600--Japan. WZ 70 JJ3]
R581
610.95--dc23
2014040526

Want or need Open Access? Brill Open offers you the choice to make your research freely accessible online in exchange for a publication charge. Review your various options on brill.com/brill-open.

Typeface for the Latin, Greek, and Cyrillic scripts: "Brill". See and download: brill.com/brill-typeface.

ISBN 978-90-04-31459-7 (paperback, 2015)
ISBN 978-90-04-28544-6 (hardback, 2015)
ISBN 978-90-04-28545-3 (e-book, 2015)

Contents

Contributors

Susan L. Burns
is Associate Professor of History and East Asian Languages and Civilizations
at the University of Chicago. Her work focuses on the late Tokugawa period to
the end of Meiji Japan. Her first book, *Before the Nation*, examined the
kokugaku discourses of the late Tokugawa period and explored how nativist
scholars constructed Japan's cultural and social identity. Her research also
investigates the medical culture of the nineteenth century and analyzes the
impact of the rise of "Western medicine" and public health upon conceptions
of the body and subjecthood. She also studies the intersection of medical and
legal discourse in the formation of modern conceptions of gender.

Benjamin A. Elman
is Gordon Wu '58 Professor of Chinese Studies at Princeton University. He
works at the intersection of several fields, including history, philosophy,
literature, religion, economics, politics, and science. His ongoing interest is in
rethinking how the history of East Asia has been told in the West as well as in
China, Japan, and Korea. He is currently studying cultural interactions in East
Asia during the eighteenth century, in particular the impact of Chinese
classical learning, medicine, and natural studies on Tokugawa Japan and
Chosŏn Korea.

Asaf Goldschmidt
is currently the Chair of the East Asian Department at Tel Aviv University. His
research focuses on the history of medicine during the Song dynasty (960–
1279). Currently he is working on two projects: the history of the Imperial
Pharmacy in China, 1076–1600; and the history of medical case histories and
medical practice during the Song dynasty.

Angela Ki Che Leung
received her doctoral degree in history at the Ecole des hautes études en
sciences sociales, Paris, and became a research fellow at the Academia Sinica
of Taibei in 1982. She has also taught in the history department of National
Taiwan University. She left Taiwan in 2008 to take up the position of Chair
Professor in History at the Chinese University of Hong Kong. In January 2011,
she became the Director and Chair Professor of the Hong Kong Institute for
the Humanities and Social Sciences of the University of Hong Kong. She also

holds the Joseph Needham–Philip Mao Professorship in Chinese History, Science, and Civilization. She was elected Academician of the Academia Sinica in 2010.

Federico Marcon

is Assistant Professor of Japanese History at Princeton University. He specializes in early modern Japan and has completed a forthcoming work, *The Knowledge of Nature and the Nature of Knowledge in Early Modern Japan,* in which he reconstructs the development of a field of natural history in the Tokugawa period. He is now working on a second book project provisionally entitled "What Money Could Buy: A Social History of Money in Early Modern Japan."

Mayanagi Makoto

is Professor of the History of Chinese Science in the College of Humanities at Ibaraki University. His specialty is the history of medicine in China and Japan, along with its philology and history of cultural interactions. His ongoing interests include how Japan absorbed Chinese medicine and refashioned it in terms of its own native style, as well as the comparative study of Korean and Vietnamese medicine between the sixteenth and eighteenth centuries.

Fabien Simonis

received his Ph.D. degree, with distinction, in 2010 from the Princeton University East Asian Studies Department for a dissertation entitled "Mad Acts, Mad Speech, and Mad People in Late Imperial Chinese Law and Medicine." He is working on two books: one on the history of Chinese medical ideas from 1100 to 1650 and one on insanity in Chinese law, medicine, and politics between 1650 and 1900. He currently resides in Dongguan, China.

Daniel Trambaiolo

received his Ph.D. degree in the History of Science Program at Princeton University in December 2013. His dissertation examines concepts of medical efficacy and their relationship to the sociological phenomenon of medical expertise in Tokugawa Japan. He is currently a postdoctoral researcher at the Hong Kong Institute for the Humanities and Social Sciences at the University of Hong Kong. He has published several articles and book chapters on the history of Japanese medicine and pharmacology between the seventeenth and nineteenth centuries and is currently revising a book manuscript tentatively titled *Ancient Texts and New Cures: Transformations of Medical Knowledge in Early Modern Japan.*

Mathias Vigouroux
is a lecturer at Zhejiang University. His research focuses on early modern
Japanese acupuncture with a particular interest in the exchange of medical
knowledge between China, Korea, and Japan and the assimilation of Chinese
acupuncture in Japan.

Rethinking the Sino-Japanese Medical Classics: Antiquarianism, Languages, and Medical Philology

Benjamin A. Elman

Be careful about reading health books. You may die of a misprint.
MARK TWAIN

∵

Based on a series of research seminars entitled "East Asia and the Early Modern World: Fresh Perspectives on Intellectual and Cultural History, 1550–1800," this second volume of our recently completed three-year (2009–2012) research cluster investigates new areas of medical history located on the margins of the present historiography of the East Asian medical classics. Using new sources, making new connections, and reexamining old assumptions, the investigators interrogate whether and why European medical modernity is an appropriate standard for delineating the modern fate of East Asia's medical classics. We have found that the exceptional importance of early modern Europe in the history of modern medicine should not be used to gloss over the equally distinctive developments in East Asia.

The essays on the history of medicine in China and Japan in this volume are written by highly regarded and accomplished junior and senior scholars. All the research is original. Each essay has something important to contribute to knowledge about a central, yet still incompletely understood dynamics of East Asian medicine, namely, the relationship between medical texts, medical practice, and practitioner identity. This volume advances our knowledge about the ways in which, through the compilation and creative rereading of texts, physicians and scholars packaged learned medical knowledge, especially how they addressed the history of different genres of texts and the ways in which textual knowledge was put into practice. The essays in this volume are especially valuable for directing our attention to the movement of medical texts between different polities and cultures of early modern East Asia, especially China and Japan. Of particular interest are the interactions, similarities, and differences

© KONINKLIJKE BRILL NV, LEIDEN, 2015 | DOI 10.1163/9789004285453_002

among medical thinkers across East Asia, who shared a similar corpus of texts yet developed divergent interpretations of the same published works. We hope this volume will be of interest and value to scholars of East Asian medical history and anthropology, as well as to scholars of medicine in other cultures who value comparative perspectives.

Based on the volume's contributions, we propose to use "philology" initially as an umbrella term for any and all activities involving the study, deployment, or evaluation of ideas contained in classical texts. The kinds of things that medical writers historically did with texts ranged widely, from historical linguistic research into ambiguous terms, to collating topically arranged anthologies of excerpts from earlier medical writings, to what could bluntly be called "proof-texting" (a doctor's empirical experience tells him that such and such a formula works for such and such a disease, and then he searches through the literature to find a textual source to legitimate his practice).

If we were to group all our findings simply under the rubric of "philology," however, we would miss the opportunity to analyze, compare, and contrast the many different, and sometimes contradictory, things that literate practitioners did with texts. At the very least, we also need a more deliberate discussion of the term "philology" and its relation to the different kinds of text-related activities we see in this volume. For example, we can also draw a clearer and more productive distinction between "classicism" as an antiquarian orientation and "philology" as a specific epistemological strategy for identifying the facts/truths in a classic. Hence, we acknowledge that there are many faces of "philology" at work in our volume.

In the essays by Mathias Vigouroux, Susan Burns, Federico Marcon, and Angela Ki Che Leung, for instance, a different set of associations emerges, and at first sight "languages and philology" would seem to be a more natural and sufficient match for our subject, and thus obviate any extended discussion of "medicine and philology." However, the other essays, by Asaf Goldschmidt, Fabien Simonis, Daniel Trambaiolo, and Mayanagi Makoto, are more informed by a medical philology, which implies first of all a working with texts, with terms, with grammatical structures, with chronologies and contexts. Philology is the basis of an adequate and meaningful translation of texts from one language into another, from one (ancient) time into the "present," from one culture into another—such as from Chinese into Japanese, and vice versa. In our medical fields, philology involves issues such as the use of anachronistic contemporary terms in the interpretation of ancient medical concepts. Philology thus allows us to address the changing meaning of the same term, often reflecting well-known metaphors in the source language that are transposed to the target language. Although each essay touches on the reliability of received texts, some of the contributors to this volume are closer to the pursuit of language, while others roam more widely into philology.

The volume as a whole communicates a sense of cohesiveness that revolves around both the firsthand uses of language for medicine and the secondhand tools of philology needed to master the medical classics. While the title of the book and my introduction may suggest that the volume is currently configured in large part as a study of "philology and medicine," I feel justified in saying that the term "philology" is used so broadly in this volume that its explanatory power legitimately carries over to antiquarian language. While typologizing the wide range of text- or language-related activities in these very rich essays, the reader may wonder whether "philology" is the best word to describe the overall contents of the volume, but I think we can make a good argument for retaining this term. Moreover, by way of global comparison, philology was certainly relevant to what our discussants Heinrich von Staden and Anthony Grafton told us ancient and Renaissance European medical writers were also doing: (1) revising, (2) retranslating, and (3) improving the quality of the Latin of the Western classics of medicine. We can see that these goals were also appropriate to the aims of early modern antiquarian and modern Chinese and Japanese medical writers.

Once we consider that the scope and magnitude of the textualization of medical knowledge in East Asia since antiquity enhanced its transmission and translation across space and time via manuscripts copied by scribes, then the role of philology in decoding these texts also jumps out at us. The ancient and medieval textualization of the medical classics, case histories, and medical compendia all climaxed with the advent of the Song dynasty (960–1279) state and the diffusion of commercial printing throughout China. While printing enhanced the velocity of the transmission of medical writings across space and time for over a millennium, the new technology also introduced many new destabilizing forces, as Mark Twain's maxim above quietly suggests: How to choose physicians? How to choose medical texts? How to ferret out mistakes in those texts? How do we know which texts have been forged or which versions of the medical classics deserve higher ranking?

Medical philologists, often as antiquarians of language, led the search for better and more reliable texts. Often they contended that the medical lessons of the ancients had been wrongly transmitted via manuscripts and poorly inherited by printed editions such that a systematic and corrosive form of textual purification was necessary to restore the original meanings of medical doctrines and to reproduce the recommended medical recipes accurately. As some of the essays in this volume will show, medical philology lay at the heart of East Asian debates concerned with the alleged theoretical priority of the concepts (*qi,* yin and yang, Five Phases, etc.) informing the *Yellow Emperor's Inner Canon* (*Huangdi neijing* 皇帝內經) and the concrete herbal and mineral prescriptions (Ch. *bencao,* J. *honzō* 本草) delineated in the *Treatise on Cold Damage Disorders* (*Shanghan lun* 傷寒論).

In particular, the textual vicissitudes associated with the *Treatise on Cold Damage Disorders* alert us to the changing nature of medical knowledge in early modern East Asian medicine. Considered "the foundational text of pharmacotherapy in East Asia," according to Volker Scheid and others, the *Treatise* was printed since the Song in the shadow of the *Yellow Emperor's Inner Canon.* In medieval times, it circulated, if at all, in fragments among a limited association of practitioners. After 1065, the text was more widely disseminated by the Song imperial government in a state-sponsored edition, which assumed the status of a medical classic in its own right. Because of its textual inscrutability, physicians and scholars perennially debated how to employ its formulas and methods. Despite the Treatise's medical instructions for therapy, these were difficult to fathom without extensive background knowledge. Physicians used it both to affirm and to critique tradition. That is why a recent medical history project "employs these tensions and contradictions as a method for uncovering [its] changing 'epistemic virtues'—ways of embodying effective clinical practice—across East Asia from the Song to the present."[1]

We learned at our meetings that ancient Greek, Roman, and Ayurvedic medical history was very similar in its search for a perfect philology to slice through medical confusion. Von Staden, Grafton, and Shigehisa Kuriyama made clear in their comments that in the search for central medical discourses, the civilizations of the ancient Mediterranean and the Indian Ocean were suffused with debates between center and local medical traditions and similarly were trapped between state and elite support of specific traditions, which had metamorphosed into reified "schools" of medical learning and practice. "Galen's corpus" represented as much of a collage of medical statements used in multiple forms as did what we will call, following Fabien Simonis, the "Danxi 丹溪 synthesis" in China, Japan, and Korea. In each version of the "great" tradition, physicians retained or excised medical accounts that they considered "allies" or "enemies" of their current concerns.

Philology thus represented a double-edged sword that probed languages and texts across the globe. In early modern China, Japan, and Korea, the mul-

---

1   See http://www.westminster.ac.uk/eastmedicine/projects/transnational-history for the Transnational History Project entitled "Interpreting Zhang Zhongjing: The *Treatise on Cold Damage* as a Window on Changing Epistemic Formations in East Asian Medicine," organized by Volker Scheid at the University of Westminster, London.

tiple defenses of and attacks on the medical classics as the interpretive products of allies or enemies became de rigueur. The medical classics and their
formidable pages of commentary in imperial China required philologists to
sort things out and anoint the victor. They brought Zhang Zhongjing 張仲景
(150–219) and the alleged original form of his *Treatise on Cold Damage Disorders* back to life, just as Roman philologists restored Galen (130–200) as the
true inheritor of a medical methodology whose origins vis-à-vis Hippocrates
(ca. 460–370 BCE) were challenged in each generation.[2]

The essays below are presented chronologically to highlight the historical
evolution of East Asian medical traditions in light of ancient classical traditions and their postclassical reverberations throughout the early modern era,
1400–1850. The spotlight will be on China and Japan during an era when "ancients" and "moderns" clashed over the modernity of tradition and the misuses
of the medical canon. Unfortunately, an essay on the place of the *Treatise on
Cold Damage Disorders* in Chosŏn Korean medical discourse by Soyoung Suh,
which was presented at the final conference, was published elsewhere. Despite
this omission, the close interaction between early modern Japan and China in
medical terms may surprise many readers, but East Asian medical interactions
with Korea (both Korea-China and Korea-Japan) were also prevalent. Medical
philologists in East Asia may have worked through the "same" medical classics,
but they had to rip their way through generations of regional and local medical
commentaries, which they were forced to reassess, before they could grapple
with the classics themselves.

A related question bedeviling the editor is whether the current chronological structure of the volume is the most effective way to highlight the connections between the essays. If there were an identifiable historical trajectory,
with different stages or developments, which was illustrated definitively by the
different essays, then a chronological presentation would be the obvious
choice. The essays themselves, however, do not unearth an obvious historical
pattern of development. The contributors move from topic to topic, and region
to region, as well as through time. Thus, it might have been more productive to
group the essays thematically in terms of the things that people did with
texts—for example, conducting research to authenticate, verify, or standardize
textual knowledge; researching the causes of ailments to develop new therapies; publishing texts as an act of connoisseurship and bibliophilia; creating
new textual genres to embody new forms of knowledge; and so on. But this attention to topical organization also proved unsatisfactory. It undercut what
little chronology there was to hold the essays together in a historical grid. The

---

2   Nutton 1989; Lonie 1978.

essays by Goldschmidt and Trambaiolo, for example, tackled important issues in a well-defined historical context, while those of Simonis and Vigoroux attempted to trace change over several centuries.

Another issue was coherency. For example, the lack of any attention to Korea and Vietnam was problematic—given the East Asian theme of the volume. Initially, we included a chapter by Dominik Wujastyk (University of Vienna) entitled "Classical Indian Medicine: The Manuscript Transmission of Medical Knowledge in Early Modern South Asia." Although it led to fruitful discussion at the meetings, the written essay proved to be an outlier, since it was not clearly focused on the issues of philology or language, or even on East Asia. Rather, it addressed South Asian manuscripts as material objects. A longer version of the work will be published elsewhere.

One item of useful comparison that did come out of the discussion of South Asia, however, was as noted above that Song China had developed a vibrant print culture in the tenth century, almost five centuries before the Gutenberg press got going in early modern Mainz. Wujastyk noted, surprisingly, that Indian savants, scribes, and physicians never turned their backs on the importance of the manuscript in cultural production, and the dissemination of knowledge, especially medical learning, remained the work of scribes. Euclid's *Elements*, for instance, was dutifully copied and recopied for centuries in India until the nineteenth century. Similarly, we find that in medieval Japan, 1200–1600, manuscript copying by scribes was the rule, except for the publication of the Buddhist canon.[3]

Not until the Japanese wars with Ming China and Korea in the 1590s did print culture appeal to ever more secular Japanese elites. Printing was no longer simply window dressing for aristocrats or karmic good works for Zen monks printing the Tripitaka. The value of "letters" amid the pervasive illiteracy of medieval society in Japan and India made learning grammar the first step for upwardly mobile students, who were drawn to literary culture via Sanskrit in India or classical Chinese in Japan. In turn, the Japanese and Indian social and cultural elites valued the classical teacher and hired him to train their young. By opening their own schools and preparing their own textbooks, classical teachers also became the agents of language transmission and the civilizing process. Because grammar built upon memorization in a classical education, students had to master many technical rules. Since the grammarian controlled access to the classical language, his profession was embedded in the shared life of the elite. Sanskrit, because of its cosmopolitanism, and classical Chinese read in Japanese (*kanbun*) were each a useful measure of classical success be-

---

3   Kornicki 1998; Lurie 2011.

cause they worked so well and smoothly—unlike the allegedly "vulgar" vernacular language of the marketplace, or so it was claimed.[4]

Grammarians taught the forms of classical, medical, and literary analysis, and conceptual categories inherited from the past in China were now reproduced in Japan; some grammarians even taught colloquial Chinese. Japan, like India, could manage this flowering of medical knowledge via manuscripts until 1650. Thereafter, the Japanese developed an influential print culture rivaling China's in secular scope. In India, the rise of the colonial regime and its printing technology eventually took priority over the maintenance of manuscript copying in Sanskrit and Urdu during the Moghul dynasty.[5]

Chapter 2: Asaf Goldschmidt (Tel Aviv University), "Reasoning with Cases: The Transmission of Clinical Medical Knowledge in Twelfth-Century Song China"

Asaf Goldschmidt focuses on Song dynasty physicians in his essay rather than the medical classics per se. He recontextualizes the medical classics by linking them with the role of manuals and textbooks in the temporal transmission of medical knowledge. In particular, Goldschmidt emphasizes the Song reappearance of ancient indigenous knowledge via Xu Shuwei 許叔微 (1079–1154), who gave priority to the *Treatise on Cold Damage Disorders* rather than the *Yellow Emperor's Inner Canon*. At a time when Song imperial editions of the medical classics were formally compiled by state scholars, the *Treatise on Cold Damage Disorders* represented a significant philological problem for the compilers, who tried to read into its southern-based curing recipes a theoretical framework derived from the northern traditions of the *Inner Canon*.

For Goldschmidt, Xu Shuwei represents a case study of the interaction of the medical canon and doctrinal issues, which together impacted on his clinical practice during the transition from the Northern to the Southern Song. In particular, Xu tried to facilitate the recovery of "ancient medicine" (*guyi* 古醫) in Song times, an agenda more common in later dynasties. Why in the Song? We know that the medical editions published by the Song government were facilitated by the expansion of print culture from 1000 to 1250. In particular, drugs were the focus of state-sponsored works printed for mass consumption in the 970s–990s. Later, in the 1020s–1030s, the government concentrated on publishing medical classics, followed by continued revisions of the classics in

---

4   Elman 2008.
5   Cf. Kaster 1988.

the 1050s–1060s to unify their doctrinal and clinical contents, which paralleled the classical statecraft consensus that Wang Anshi 王安石 (1021–1086) sought to establish.

In 1086, however, pervasive epidemics forced Song physicians to address new medical challenges and spurred a modest revival of the *Treatise on Cold Damage Disorders*. The goal of Xu Shuwei's medical trilogy, for example, was to reeducate people about the *Treatise* as a practical handbook for curative techniques. Xu was reacting to his own personal tragedy of 1090, when the epidemics claimed his mother and father. He criticized the practical flaws in the annotations of the medical classics then available and blamed the Song medical editions for overly theorizing the *Treatise* while neglecting practical clinical knowledge. For a Ming, Qing, or Tokugawa physician, as we will see in later essays, such criticism would have been de rigueur, but during the Song, Xu had little impact, and his books were virtually lost. Not until the Qianlong-Jiaqing era (1736–1820) would there be a Qing dynasty revival of Xu's medical trilogy in a more welcoming age.

Chapter 3: Fabien Simonis (Independent Scholar), "Illness, Texts, and 'Schools' in Danxi Medicine: A New Look at Chinese Medical History from 1320 to 1800"

Fabien Simonis takes us from the era of Song physicians after the epidemics and their contending medical views to the great fourteenth-century medical syncretism, which he appropriately calls the "Danxi 丹溪 synthesis." The centrality of Zhu Zhenheng (1282–1358), honorifically named Danxi, for Chinese, Japanese, and Korean medicine from 1350 until 1600 has been poorly understood until recently because later accounts downplayed the synthesis and explained medical trends since the Song in terms of competing "schools" of medical learning. Especially egregious in this vein of "splitting" rather than "lumping" was the account by the influential compilers of the medical books included in the Qianlong Imperial Library. The latter split the history of medicine in China into northern and southern "schools." That said, however, the goal of syncretism (*zhezhong* 折中) implied a form of critical assessment when it was also accompanied by a significant degree of historical research or attempts to validate the source texts. Danxi's synthesis separated the wheat from the chaff, saved the former, and tossed the latter on the dustbin of medical history.

One unique characteristic of the Danxi synthesis was the role that Zhang Zhongjing, the ancient author of the *Treatise on Cold Damage Disorders*, played in the Song-Yuan-Ming reworking of the *Treatise* into one of the medical classics. Zhang's own notion of illness, for instance, was de-emphasized in the Danxi synthesis and reinvented as part of the synthesis Danxi envisioned. The Danxi version of Zhang Zhongjing emphasized the latter's views on the uniqueness of the illnesses he faced in the era of post-Han epidemics and his flexible art of prescription to deal with the disease symptoms that he identified. The Danxi synthesis thus served as an intertextual composition that drew on citations selectively appropriated to suit an eclectic appraisal and to reconcile conflicting doctrines.

Liu Chun 劉純 (1340–1412), for example, prepared a "best passages" digest of Zhang Zhongjing's bequeathed writings. Lou Ying 樓英 (1320–1400) wrote up a summa of Zhang's views that systematized the *Treatise* and reconciled it with the various approaches cited in the Danxi corpus of medical classics and handbooks. Like Zhu Xi's 朱熹 (1130–1200) grand synthesis for Way Learning (*daoxue* 道學), Zhu Danxi provided the textualized glue that held the Song-Yuan-Ming medical consensus together based on Way Learning cosmology and contemporary medical practices drawing on Zhang Zhongjing's recipes. Wang Lun 王綸 (1453–1510) classified a stable set of therapies, which he retheorized in light of "ministerial fire" (*huo* 火). He then added the need to restrain human desires as a required therapy to deal with heat factor illnesses. But this shift represented in part a tactical retreat from Danxi to Zhang Zhongjing and the *Treatise*, which had included the treatment of warm factor illnesses in its repertoire.

The reinvention of the so-called "Song-Yuan-Ming masters" as archrivals by their archaist opponents after 1600, however, made it seem as if the Song-Yuan-Ming masters had never included Zhang Zhongjing in their synthesis. By rejecting them as uncritical lumpers of the medical classics, the champions of ancient medicine in China, Japan, and Korea split off the *Treatise on Cold Damage Disorders* from the Danxi synthesis and heralded Zhang's therapeutics of "ancient recipes" (*gufang*) instead. Zhang Zhongjing replaced Zhu Danxi in the medical hierarchy, a revival that later raised up lesser voices from the Song such as Xu Shuwei to positions of medical eminence.

By 1600, a division between "fire depletion" and "*qi* replenishing" as desirable therapies displaced the milder and less interventionist Danxi synthesis. Rather than syncretism, the ancient-medicine radicals favored a notion of competing schools. The ancients—that is, Zhang Zhongjing and his *Treatise*—were resurrected at the expense of the Song-Yuan-Ming "Danxi synthesis" of medical learning. Simonis demonstrates that the early modern disappearance of the Danxi partisan's notion of a synthesis should not be taken at face value. A new synthesis was in the works during the seventeenth and eighteenth

centuries, which built on the apparent irreconcilable tensions among competing views of ancient medicine.

Chapter 4: Daniel Trambaiolo (University of Hong Kong), "Ancient Texts and New Medical Ideas in Eighteenth-Century Japan"

Daniel Trambaiolo carries the medical story beyond China to include early
modern Japan. He describes how the philological turn based on newly discovered medieval manuscripts in Tokugawa times (1600–1867) empowered ancient medicine in light of the clash between old medical classics and new
ideas. The polarity between the *Treatise on Cold Damage Disorders* and the *Yellow Emperor's Inner Canon* pitted the Danxi synthesis against critical philology
in Japan as well. By reassessing the medical classics via case histories that focused on a physician's own experience, the latter textually discredited the
Danxi synthesis and linked ancient learning (*kogaku* 古學) with ancient formulas (*kohō* 古方). The new classicism of the Tokugawa era represented a
medical and scholarly intersection, which empowered the recovery of ancient
medical learning and the undoing of the Danxi synthesis. Zhu Xi's classical
orthodoxy faced a similar onslaught of the "ancients" versus the "moderns" in
the eighteenth century in Qing China and Tokugawa Japan.

The rising social status of Japanese physicians after 1650 challenged existing
social hierarchies. In a futile reply, Tokugawa classicists such as Itō Jinsai 伊藤
仁斎 (1627–1705) and Dazai Shundai 太宰春台 (1680–1747) tried to lower the
boom on such pretensions by attacking the nouveau riche origins of many of
their peers. The divisions between samurai physicians and commoner classical
doctors took over a century to work out and informed the efforts by mainstream upholders of the Danxi synthesis to try to counter the radical physicians who championed Zhang Zhongjing's ancient medical legacy. Jinsai's
disdain for the commoner physicians parading around as highbrow Confucians was social and not intellectual. Both samurai and commoners spurned
the magico-religious traditions of nativist medicine. Jinsai's own commoner
students called for the Confucianization of the medical tradition based on the
new philology of ancient texts, however. The philologically suspect *Yellow Emperor's Inner Canon* lost its place of eminence in the flood of medical collations
and studies bringing the so-called "original" version of the *Treatise on Cold
Damage Disorders* back to life.

Trambaiolo points to Yamawaki Tōyō's 山脇東洋 (1705–1762) "return to antiquity" (*fuko* 復古) as an example of the cutting edge of medical learning in
the eighteenth century. Yamawaki's focus on anatomy predated the more

ballyhooed Sugita Genpaku 杉田玄白 (1733–1817), who linked new medical trends with Dutch Learning (*rangaku* 蘭学). Loyal more to changing Chinese medical findings, Yamawaki saw the body holistically and appealed to the unity of the ancients and moderns (*kokin* 古今) in addressing a new anatomy. He replaced the *Yellow Emperor's Inner Canon's* theoretical models with a view of the body informed jointly by a philological and an anatomical focus. Sugita would later leap over Yamawaki to stress the importance of anatomy in Dutch medicine and gain most of the credit that Yamawaki deserved in this vein.

Another of the eighteenth-century archaists, Yoshimasu Tōdō 吉益東洞 (1702–1773), linked his therapeutic empiricism to language skepticism. I should add that his disciple Murai Kinzan 村井琴山 (1733–1815), for example, presented philological proof that identifications of specific medical recipes in the *Yellow Emperor's Inner Canon* were based on mistaken understanding of the rhymes. By combining philology with empirical research, Yoshimasu dismissed the yin-yang traditions of Daoist physicians and the "illness identification focus" of Confucian doctors as convenient explanatory devices that tried to determine causes based on symptoms.

The power of long-taken-for-granted concepts to deceive physicians was Yoshimasu's starting point. He emphasized instead a "single poison" as the cause for all illness and saw the stagnation of *qi* in the body as the best way to first identify and then link symptoms to medical theory, rather than the other way around. He disallowed theory the power to overdetermine actual symptoms. For Yoshimasu, a theory should always remain focused on curing and not on reducing an illness to theoretical constructs. Like Yamawaki, Yoshimasu opposed slow and gentle nourishment in favor of activist intervention through purging. He regarded ginseng recipes, for example, as an acute therapy and not a form of repletion of the body. He also stressed medical recipes in the tradition of Zhang Zhongjing over the traditional materia medica (*honzō* 本草) associated with the Song-Yuan-Ming masters of the Danxi synthesis.

Chapter 5: Mathias Vigouroux (Zhejiang University), "The Reception of the Circulation Channels Theory in Japan (1500–1800)"

Japanese physicians reconsidered the efficacy of acupuncture, which they adapted to Japan's medical traditions. Before 1600, acupuncture was used in China, Japan, and Korea mainly as a crude surgical tool for bloodletting. There was little stress after 1600 on a pulse examination or the acupuncture channels. But Kamakura monks in Japan, ironically, favored moxibustion, of all the techniques associated with acupuncture, to stop bleeding. As with the medical learning associated with Zhang Zhongjing, the early theories of acupuncture points were not revived until the Song dynasty in China. Thereafter, Song physicians focused on the circulation channels for the *qi* and located the acupuncture points along the body affecting the flow of *qi*. They standardized the channels and numbered the points, but the impact of these Chinese-inspired innovations on medieval Japanese medicine was still minimal.

Mathias Vigouroux contends that the lack of Heian-Kamakura (900–1400) support for acupuncture was due to Japan's seclusion policy vis-à-vis China, especially during the Mongol era. After 1401, exchanges with China increased and led to the revival of acupuncture in the late sixteenth century, along with herbal medicine. In the seventeenth century, the transformation of acupuncture in Japan drew on the teachings of the Yuan physician Hua Shou 滑壽 (fl. 1340–1370). The Ashikaga physician Manase Dōsan 曲直瀬 道三 (1507–1594), for example, used Hua's textbook in 1563. Later, in 1661, a Japanese commentary for Hua's work appeared. Nevertheless, Chinese illustrations of acupuncture at the time, such as those by Wang Weiyi 王惟一 (987–1067), had little influence. In Japan, acupuncturists introduced the Dutch anatomist Willem ten Rhyne (1647–1700) to its most rudimentary techniques in the 1670s.

During the eighteenth century, however, Tokugawa physicians began to reconsider the efficacy of the circulation channels as part of the turn toward ancient medicine and Zhang Zhongjing's *Treatise on Cold Damage Disorders*. In contrast, there were no significant changes or developments in acupuncture during the "high Qing" period in China. Hua Shou's tradition of fourteen channels was virtually lost. In Japan, Ishizaka Sōtetsu 石坂宗哲 (1770–1841) associated the circulation channels with the blood and nervous systems, which Japanese had assimilated since 1800 as part of Dutch Learning. Ishizaka also used anatomy to recover the methods of acupuncture by stressing the dichotomy between conscious nerves and transport nerves. This mapping of acupuncture onto the nervous system, and associating *qi* with the circulation of blood, produced a flowering of acupuncture in Japan in the nineteenth century that was not matched in Qing China until Chinese students studied in Meiji Japan after 1895.

Chapter 6: Susan L. Burns (University of Chicago), "A Village Doctor and the *Treatise on Cold Damage Disorders* (*Shanghan lun* 傷寒論): Medical Theory / Medical Practice in Late Tokugawa Japan"

Susan Burns takes us deeper into the world of traditional Japanese medicine by introducing us to a village doctor in northeastern Japan in the early nineteenth century. At this level of analysis we can see the wide impact that the revival of ancient medicine had and the pervasive turn toward Zhang Zhongjing's medical teachings that occurred at the local level far from the great cities of Kyoto, Osaka, and Edo. Nanayama Jundō 七山順道 (fl. 1818–1868) produced 225 medical case records from 1824 to 1833, which he included among his library of medical classics and contemporary works. His professional, intellectual, and social worlds allow us to see the interlocking processes of the medicalization of illness, the commodification of medicine, and the social networks that physicians formed in the last decades of the Tokugawa shogunate.

Moved by the parallels he saw between the epidemics recorded by Zhang Zhongjing in the *Treatise on Cold Damage Disorders* and the epidemics of his own time, Nanayama was one of the fifty physicians who prepared commentaries for the *Treatise* between 1790 and 1830. Altogether, the Tokugawa era produced 120 medical works on Zhang Zhongjing and the *Treatise*. Like others who turned to the *Treatise*, Nanayama saw in Zhang a voice of opposition to the *Yellow Emperor's Inner Canon* and its overtheorization as part of the Danxi synthesis. In his medical case records, Nanyama stressed diagnostics for treatment that included examinations of pulse variations, an emphasis on practical findings over textual knowledge, and a stress on observation and experience. The cases represented a new form of medical writing, which had begun in Ming China when many Chinese physicians in South China turned to the *Treatise* as a guide for dealing with epidemics. From 1600 to 1800, Zhang Zhongjing penetrated the vibrant world of medical practice in Japan down to the village level.

Chapter 7: Federico Marcon (Princeton University), "*Honzōgaku* after *Seibutsugaku*: Traditional Pharmacology as Antiquarianism after the Institutionalization of Modern Biology in Early Meiji Japan"

Federico Marcon's chapter on new forms of natural knowledge carries us into the late Tokugawa and early Meiji periods when Dutch Learning in Japan was surpassed by a wave of Westernization in all things Japanese, especially medicine and materia medica (*honzōgaku* 本草學). The emerging Tokugawa market economy was both a cause and an enabling factor in the growing link between herbal pharmaceuticals and economic growth. Local trade and commerce commoditized herbal medicines in Japan and also contributed to an interregional commodity trade in medicines between China, Japan, and Korea and then globally with Europe, the Americas, and Southeast Asia. The exchange of cultural goods across the now more fluid social classes also contributed to the upward social circulation of Western-trained physicians, who achieved very high status as wealthy members of Japanese society.

Marcon notes that the 1830s marked the time when the instrumental value of *honzō* for Japanese agriculture became a key measure of the importance of modern medicines and natural science in the Japanese economy. The very notion of *honzōgaku* as materia medica became suspect in an age when Western medicine was deemed superior to all aspects of the *kanpō* 漢方 traditions of medication. Just as Western-trained physicians delegitimized the medical classics in a frenzy of Westernization, so too they disenfranchised the ancient medical traditions of the Tokugawa era. Meiji elites routinely branded the Tokugawa era as a "failed" era based on Western paradigms that replaced native values—so much so that we will see in Mayanagi's concluding chapter that Meiji Japanese willingly sold off their traditional medical texts to still-interested Chinese and curious Europeans.

Marcon explains that the Japanese rethinking of *honzōgaku* in the Tokugawa era according to the standards of modern medicine meant that many aspects of *honzōgaku* could be assimilated to Western natural science as a nativist form of "natural history." But those aspects of *honzōgaku* that could not be naturalized as Western remained associated with what was now considered the "failed" *kanpō* tradition. Ironically, the turn from *Kanpō* to Western medicine made the most of the *honzōgaku* part of *Kanpō*. The old materia medica were superimposed on the new framework of Western medical therapies.

The adaptation of *honzōgaku* practices and theories to the Western botanical sciences of Linnaeus also diminished the local status of *kanpō* physicians in the late nineteenth century. The earlier Confucian scholarly links to the new Tokugawa naturalists helped to increase the role of the Meiji state in medicine, but adherents of ancient medical practices such as Asada Sōhaku 浅田 宗伯 (1815–1894), for example, were seen as relics of the past, anachronisms in a new age. The *kanpō* revival in the 1890s represented a reaction against the early Meiji processes of over-Westernization. *Honzōgaku* specialists such as Mori Risshi 森立之 (1807–1885) mobilized the remnants of the *Kanpō* and *honzōgaku* constituencies in 1891, but the damage had been done. Japanese traditional medicine, like traditional medicine in China, was now second class.

Chapter 8: Angela Ki Che Leung (University of Hong Kong), "Japanese Medical Texts in Chinese on *Kakké* in the Tokugawa and Early Meiji Periods"

Our concluding essays by Angela Ki Che Leung and Mayanagi Makoto address explicitly the flow of texts and medical knowledge between China and Japan. Their essays are particularly valuable contributions and a nice counter to the earlier chapters, which take up either China or Japan. Angela Leung's chapter, for example, retraces another important aspect of medical philology in Japan from the Tokugawa to the Meiji period—namely, the reformulation and re-definition of premodern diseases into their modern forms.

On the basis of Western biomedical concepts circa 1900, beriberi was de-fined as an illness caused by the deficiency of vitamin B1. In Japan, the disease had been called *kakké* 腳氣 since classical times and was still defined in the early Meiji period as a *kanpō* illness caused by a Wind toxin. Similarly, the dis-ease was known as *jiaoqi* 腳氣 in late imperial China, on the basis of the clas-sical etiological analysis of leg-wind: the pathogens of Damp and Wind entered by the lower limbs. *Jiaoqi* was surprisingly ignored by late imperial medical texts except for a couple mentioning an eruption of cases in Guangzhou (Can-ton) early in the nineteenth century. Modern Chinese often had to rely on Meiji *kanpō* texts to interpret the old disease called *jiaoqi*.

Belief in illnesses that were caused by nutrient deficiencies had little follow-ing in Asia before 1930. *Kakké* had a flexible therapeutics in Japan, however. On the basis of classical *kanpō* concepts of the disorder, it was further interpreted as a disease of the prosperous, which also attacked the young and able-bodied due to their unhealthy diets and lifestyles. For this reason it preyed on the new class of the urban rich in Japan—hedonistic and decadent—who were depen-dent on their rice diet. Doctors applied regimes of purging and replenishing for therapeutics, methods that were based on traditional Chinese medical classics on *jiaoqi*. The toxin was controlled through depletion blockage, and then acu-puncture was applied along with replenishing via the use of herbal prescrip-tions. Indeed, *kanpō* etiology and therapeutics included enough mention of some sort of bodily deficiency that this aspect influenced Western biomedical views of beriberi, but it was still seen as a distinctly Japanese disease.

Kanpō also informed Patrick Manson's (1844–1922) view of tropical medi-cine that he developed over three decades in residence as a consular physician in Taiwan and Xiamen (Amoy). Leung concludes that beriberi, *kakké*, and *ji-aoqi* were not just three names for the same disease. Each was conceptualized differently and included different expectations for both the cause and the effect of the illness. Even though the emergence of the biomedical category of a "vitamin deficiency disease" eventually dominated after the 1930s, the term "beriberi" never fully translated the meanings of *kakké* or *jiaoqi*, which had to be understood in their historical and cultural contexts.

Chapter 9: Mayanagi Makoto (Ibaraki University), with Takashi Miura (Princeton University) and Mathias Vigouroux (Zhejiang University), "Yang Shoujing and the Kojima Family: Collection and Publication of Medical Classics"

The Meiji decline of *Kanpō* described by Marcon earlier is further elaborated by Mayanagi Makoto in our concluding chapter. Medical book hunting in Tokugawa Japan had been linked to the popularity of both the Ancient Formulas School and *kanpō* traditionalists. Through their search for medical evidence, they sought to justify their disagreements and to support their own theories. Despite the earlier links of the Edo Medical School to *kanpō* medicine, the Meiji endorsed Western medicine in the medical school as the professional standard in the 1880s and thereby disenfranchised generations of traditional practitioners. Although this policy was reversed in 1902, it came too late for precious Tokugawa medical texts that were sold off in the early Meiji period.

The late Qing diplomat Yang Shoujing 楊守敬 (1839–1915) lived in Japan from 1880 to 1884. Taking advantage of the Meiji dismantling of *Kanpō*, he obtained the Kojima 小島 family's medical collection, which had been based on three generations of practitioners/collectors who had collated many medical texts. From 1648 to the end of the Tokugawa period, many members of the Kojima family had been shogun physicians. At its height, the Kojima family owned over one thousand Chinese medical titles, and they also preserved seventy-eight rare Japanese books—thirty-five of which are now in the National Palace Museum in Taibei. At one time the Kojima family had preserved 646 rare books on medicine from China and Japan.

With the help and involvement of Mori Tatsuyuki, Yang Shoujing purchased 30,000 *juan* in 1880–1881 from the Kojima family's widow, after her husband, Kojima Shōkei 小島尚絅 (1839–1880), lost his medical academy position after the Meiji Restoration and died in poverty in 1880. After his own death in 1915, Yang's books wound up in the National Library in Beijing by 1929 and, by 1933, in Nanjing. Of these, 1,724 were medical volumes that are now in Taibei at the National Palace Museum. The decline of *Kanpō* in the early Meiji period had dragged down with it the rich Tokugawa collections particularly in Edo, Kyoto, and Osaka. Many of the rare books perished or made their way via opportunistic book buyers such as Yang Shoujing to China, where they contributed to the revival of traditional Chinese medicine in the 1920s and 1930s.

Republication of many of Yang's volumes in Wuchang and Shanghai later made these Tokugawa medical texts available in China, and they were restored to Japanese university libraries thereafter. It was the end of an era, however, as traditional medicine in China and traditional medicine in Japan struggled to maintain their shared medical identities amid the Sino-Japanese animosities of the twentieth century. Philologists of medical texts were less and less likely to be actual medical practitioners, where once they always had been. The modern history of medicine as a discipline effectively displaced the practical relevance of ancient medicine in the contemporary world.

• • •

The individual essays in this volume, one by one, tell us the story of a proud millennial medical tradition in East Asia that peaked from 1600 to 1800. In modern China, Japan, Korea, and Southeast Asia, however, the raison d'être of traditional medicine in Shanghai, Tokyo, Seoul, and Hanoi was increasingly challenged and placed on the defensive in dealing with the global cholera, typhoid, plague, and influenza epidemics of the nineteenth and early twentieth centuries, which the more activist epidemiological tactics of modern medicine handled more successfully.

The overall contribution of this volume suggests, however, that the so-called "failure" narrative for traditional medicine in East Asia was a temporary and premature manufacture. We can no longer view traditional medicine as a field that just focused on itself and thereby reproduced itself as irrational superstition. The "warm factor illnesses" of Zhang Zhongjing, for example, have been successfully assimilated with the modern versions of "tropical medicine" that Manson and others first began to understand while serving as Euro-American physicians in Xiamen (Amoy) and Danshui (Tamsui). The received narrative of medical history in East Asia is no longer simply a tale of the vices of traditional medicine in contrast to the "miracle drugs" of the "West." As microbial resistance to our former "wonder drugs" continues to expand, we are increasingly brought back to lifestyle, balanced diet, and herbal remedies to help alleviate illness and create wellness, that is, "preserving life" (*yangsheng* 養生).[6]

---

6   Cf. DiMoia 2013. See also Elman 2005, chap. 11.

In closing, I would again like to thank Heinrich von Staden (Institute for Advanced Study), Anthony Grafton (Princeton University), and Shigehisa Kuriyama (Harvard University) for their participation as discussants and commentators at the February 10, 2012, workshop upon which this conference volume is based. Their comments influenced many of the chapters in this volume, including this one. I also wish to acknowledge the contributions of Constanze Magdalene Güthenke (then at Princeton, now at Oxford University), Soyoung Suh (Dartmouth College), Pamela Smith (Columbia University), and Harold Cook (Brown University). The outside readers chosen by Brill also made numerous interventions and offered many suggestions that challenged us to rethink our findings and clarify our claims.

References

DiMoia, John P. 2013. *Reconstructing Bodies: Biomedicine, Health, and Nation-Building in South Korea since 1945*. Stanford, CA: Stanford University Press.

Elman, Benjamin 2005. *On Their Own Terms: Science in China, 1550–1900*. Cambridge, MA: Harvard University Press.

———— 2008. "Sinophiles and Sinophobes in Tokugawa Japan: Politics, Classicism, and Medicine during the Eighteenth Century," *East Asian Science, Technology and Society: An International Journal* (Taiwan) 2, 1 (March): 93–121.

Kaster, Robert 1988. *Guardians of Language: The Grammarian and Society in Late Antiquity*. Berkeley: University of California Press.

Kornicki, Peter 1998. *The Book in Japan: A Cultural History from the Beginnings to the Nineteenth Century*. Leiden: E. J. Brill.

Lonie, I. M. 1978. "Cos versus Cnidus and the Historians, Part 1," *History of Science* 16 (March): 42–75.

Lurie, David 2011. *Realms of Literacy: Early Japan and the History of Writing*. Cambridge, MA: Harvard University Asia Center. Distributed by Harvard University Press.

Nutton, Vivian 1989. "Hippocrates in the Renaissance," in *Die hippokratischen Epidemien*, edited by Gerhard Baader and Rolf Winau. Stuttgart: Franz Steiner, 420–439.

CHAPTER 2

Reasoning with Cases: The Transmission of Clinical Medical Knowledge in Twelfth-Century Song China

Asaf Goldschmidt

Historians are often interested in the transmission of knowledge or, more specifically, how scholars propagate their knowledge to posterity. While there is a growing body of studies examining how medical knowledge, especially textual, has been transmitted from one culture to another or has migrated from one region to the next, less work has focused on the transmission of medical knowledge temporally, from one generation of practitioners to the next. We should remember that "transmission" is, of course, a complex and multifaceted process, especially when we are discussing physicians' clinical know-how. Transmitting the doctrines explaining the body and its functions from a master to a pupil is no easy task, but teaching the disciple how to palpate the pulse and diagnose a disorder is a whole different ordeal, especially when authors attempt to undertake this task in writing. In other words, when discussing transmission of medical knowledge, which inherently includes the transmission of medical practices as well, we have to ponder what are the most effective textual means to transmit the complete manifold of physicians' knowledge to the audience of readers.

The problem of transmitting practical knowledge concerned Chinese thinkers from early times, as we find in the *Zhuangzi*. In the story about the duke and the wheelwright, Zhuangzi discussed different modes of knowledge transmission while challenging common perceptions:

> Duke Huan was reading a book at the top of the hall, wheelwright [Bian] was chipping a wheel at the bottom of the hall. He put aside his mallet and chisel, and went up to ask Duke Huan
> "May I ask what words my lord is reading?"
> "The words of a sage."
> "Is the sage alive?"
> "He is dead."
> "In that case what my lord is reading is the dregs of the men of old, isn't it?"

© KONINKLIJKE BRILL NV, LEIDEN, 2015 | DOI 10.1163/9789004285453_003

"What business is it of a wheelwright to criticize what I read? If you can explain yourself, well and good; if not, you die."

"Speaking for myself, I see it in terms of my own work. If I chip at a wheel too slowly, the chisel slides and does not grip; if too fast, it jams and catches in the wood. Not too slow, not too fast; I feel it in the hand and respond from the heart, the mouth cannot put it into words, there is a knack in it somewhere which I cannot convey to my son and which my son cannot learn from me. This is how through my seventy years I have grown old chipping at wheels. The men of old and their untransmittable message are dead. Then what my lord is reading is the dregs of men of old, isn't it?"[1]

Zhuangzi's goal in presenting this story was probably to debunk the importance and effectiveness of language, especially written language, in transmitting knowledge. He also showed his objection to the Confucian claim that the ancients have handed down the essential knowledge on how to manage state and society. We can agree or disagree with this claim, but we do have to take into consideration the story's main point—namely, that transmitting practical know-how is problematic—since the most important aspect in transmitting medical knowledge is transmitting practical clinical knowledge and acquired experience. According to Zhuangzi, useful knowledge—the skills one acquires over years of practice in this case—cannot be transmitted by textual means. This has direct bearing on the physician's task when he attempts to pass his accumulated clinical knowledge to posterity, especially to a broader audience beyond his disciples. In other words, we have to consider the following question: Can a physician truly transmit his accumulated body of clinical knowledge, in addition to his theoretical knowledge, to his readers or is this a futile endeavor?

In this essay I will discuss a Song dynasty (960–1276) physician and his struggle to transmit his theoretical interpretation and clinical application of the doctrines included in an ancient medical canon reprinted by the Song government after virtually being out of circulation for centuries. This physician, Xu Shuwei, compiled and published a collection of his own medical case histories to achieve this goal, although from a historical perspective he may have had only little effect on his peers' medical practice and understanding of medicine. It is important to note that Xu published the first collection of a Chinese physician's personal case histories. I will outline Xu's life and work, focusing on his case histories. My claim is that he recorded and published his own case

---

1   Graham 1981, 139–140. See also Yearley 1996.

histories in order to facilitate comprehension of the newly rediscovered Cold Damage doctrines and their integration with contemporary medical practice. His book, however, soon fell out of circulation and was forgotten for two or more centuries before receiving some recognition.

Medical Cases in China

Throughout most of China's history, the recording of medical case histories was never as popular as it was in the West. In China we do not find extensive collections of physicians' case histories in medical treatises as early as the *Hippocratic Corpus* or Galen's writings.[2] Before the second millennium CE, it seems that Chinese physicians did not perceive medical case histories as an essential literary medium with which to hand down their clinical knowledge to the next generation. This may be due to the fact that the majority of physicians until the Song dynasty acquired their medical skills from elder physicians who were either family members transmitting their knowledge within the family lineage or master physicians teaching handpicked disciples.[3] Acquiring medical knowledge in this manner does not make recording case histories a necessity since the disciple spends years at the teacher's side learning firsthand from his observations at the patients' bedside. This changed during the Song dynasty and even more so during the Ming, once printed medical literature became available at a relatively inexpensive price. During the Song dynasty the establishment of an imperial medical education system provided another alternative venue for obtaining medical knowledge.

In the past two decades a number of scholars have published studies focusing on the history of medical case histories in China and have concluded that it was not until the Ming dynasty (1368–1644) that physicians began to record and publish their teachers' or their own medical case histories.[4] Although we find records of medical cases before the Ming dynasty, by and large, imperial officials rather than physicians documented these cases. Accordingly, these medical cases differed from physicians' cases since they served different goals and had a different target audience. The first collection of medical case histories in China appears in the *Records of the Grand Historian* by Sima Qian (90 BCE). In chapter 105, titled "The Biographies of Bian Que and Cang Gong" (*Shiji* 扁鵲倉公列傳), the author detailed the testimony of a physician by the

---

2   Alvarez 1999, 2010; Mattern 2008.
3   Sivin 1995.
4   Hu 2009; Furth 2007a, 2007b; Cullen 2001; Grant 2003; Shi and Xiao 1994.

name of Chunyu Yi 淳于意 (215–ca. 150 BCE, also known as Cang Gong) concerning his medical training and clinical practice. Asked by the emperor to explain his medical arts, Chunyu Yi delineated where and how he obtained his medical knowledge and then provided twenty-five medical records to exemplify his superior pulse diagnoses, which, according to his account, enabled his remarkable ability to distinguish between fatal and curable diseases.[5] Approximately four hundred years later, we find additional case histories recorded for another physician, Hua Tuo 華佗 (ca. 140–208 CE), in the official histories of the Eastern Han dynasty and of the Three Kingdoms.[6] It is important to note that in both these instances imperial officials recorded the medical cases as part of the biographies of Chunyu Yi and Hua Tuo. Consequently, these records were designed, not to transmit medical knowledge to posterity, but rather to glorify the legacy and expertise of these two physicians.

Until the Song dynasty we find very few examples of case histories in surviving records; the most familiar are those by the Tang dynasty physician Sun Simiao 孫思邈 (581–682). In his monumental formulary *Essential Recipes Worth a Thousand Gold Pieces, for Urgent Need* (*Beiji qianjin yaofang* 備急千金要方), Sun included several records or anecdotes from his own experience to serve as specific examples of the efficacy of prescriptions he discusses. The number of these records is limited and they are not listed together systematically.[7] Sun's case records are essentially anecdotal and are not literary tools designed to transmit medical knowledge. It seems that Sun inserted these cases in order to illustrate or clarify specific issues relating to certain medicinal formulas but not as a literary measure to enhance the transmission of medical knowledge, since he did not include case records systematically with each of the formulas he presents.

During the Song dynasty we find for the first time medical case records bundled together in medical treatises. In the writings of two prominent physicians—Qian Yi and Xu Shuwei—we find two examples of this innovation. Their collections of cases offer detailed narratives of the clinical encounter, the doctor's diagnosis, and the herbal formula or formulas prescribed as a remedy. The first collection—twenty-five records of pediatric case histories—is included in a book supposedly authored by Qian Yi 錢乙 (ca. 1032–1113) and titled *Proven Formulas of Medicine for Small Children* (*Xiao'er yaozheng zhijue* 小兒藥證直訣). Although at first glance these case histories may seem to have

---

5   For translations, see Hsu 2010; Sivin 1995.
6   *Hou Han shu, juan* 112; *San Guo zhi, juan* 29. For translations, see DeWoskin 1983, 140–153; Mair 1994.
7   Sivin 1967.

been written by the physician Qian Yi, this is not the case; an interested third party recorded them. A grateful father of one of Qian's young patients collected success stories from other parents of Qian's patients and recorded them in a book bearing Qian Yi's name.[8] This book, though intriguing due to its emphasis on pediatrics, was not a comprehensive treatise consisting predominantly of cases handpicked by the physician. Once again, it is more a collection of stories or anecdotes illustrating the grandeur of a physician rather than a literary means to transmit knowledge. This is exactly where the recorded cases of Qian Yi and Xu Shuwei differ. The first collection was compiled by a patient's parent to glorify the skills of the physician who treated his child, whereas the second collection was compiled by Xu Shuwei himself and was designed to facilitate the transmission of knowledge to future generations. Xu's collection, aimed toward a readership of fellow experts, links together the classical doctrines of Cold Damage with contemporary clinical decision making.

It was not until the second half of the Ming dynasty that case histories emerged as a self-conscious genre of medical writing termed *yi'an* 醫案. In 1531 *The Medical Cases of Wang Ji* (also titled *Cases of the Stone Mountain, Shishan yi'an* 石山醫案) signaled a change in the focus of medical literature to case histories and was soon followed by numerous treatises. A number of studies have discussed the sudden rise in publications of case histories. Christopher Cullen claimed that the increased popularity of this genre was due to the adaptation of the judicial case format to medicine in order to promote the status and prestige of physicians and their medical lineages.[9] Joanna Grant claimed that the growing networks connecting physicians, merchants, and book publishers brought about the literary genre of *yi'an*.[10] Charlotte Furth argued that the case history as a literary genre was used to mediate the tension between canon and doctrine, on the one hand, and clinical practice, on the other. Case histories thus enabled physicians to reconcile medical "scholarly currents" in the context of one doctor's clinical preferences, thereby supporting and consolidating the lineage of practitioners associated with him.[11]

The above depiction of the history of medical case histories in China, in which prior to the Ming dynasty no physician compiled a collection of either his or his teacher's clinical records to transmit to posterity, has one significant exception. In 1132 a Song physician, Xu Shuwei 許叔微 (1079–1154), compiled and later published a collection of his medical case

---

8   Hsiung 2007, 155–156.
9   Cullen 2001, 310–322.
10   Grant 2003, 21–50.
11   Furth 2007b, 132–133.

histories—*Ninety Discussions on Cold Damage Disorders* (*Shanghan jiushi lun* 傷寒九十論). Additionally, he published several dozen case records concerning many disorders besides Cold Damage in his formulary entitled the *Original Formulary for Popular Relief* (*Puji benshi fang* 普濟本事方).[12] Furth and Cullen mention Xu Shuwei's *Ninety Discussions on Cold Damage Disorders*, but they both perceive it as an aberration, essentially dismissing it as not belonging to this genre.[13] I claim that Xu's work is and should be regarded as a collection of medical case histories despite its isolation within the Song context. Xu chose the cases he included in his book and provided both case details and an annotated discussion elaborating the doctrinal logic behind the diagnosis and the treatment. Xu authored, not an anecdotal collection of cases, but rather a pedagogical tool aimed to aid the reader in solving the mystery of diagnosing and treating Cold Damage disorders in an era when this genre of medicine was just rediscovered after years of inaccessibility to its literature.[14] Below I will discuss Xu's book and explain why he chose to utilize this innovative genre in his writings.

Unlike during the Ming dynasty, when the publication of medical case histories became an established literary genre, Xu Shuwei's book stood alone. Therefore, we must ask, why did Xu write this unique book? In other words, what was the general or medical context that prompted Xu to produce a book in a genre that had never been used before by physicians to transmit medical knowledge? I claim that a new medical environment, in which newly printed, government-sponsored, ancient medical works became widely accessible to physicians, revealed a theoretical and practical conflict between the contents of the older works and contemporary practice. I contend that Xu chose this innovative literary style in order to convey his integration of ancient and contemporary medical knowledge. In other words, he chose this literary genre as a means of transmitting both his own clinical medical knowledge and how it fit with his interpretation of newly available ancient medical knowledge concerning Cold Damage disorders. If we look at the structure of his work, as well

---

12   Sometimes this book is found under the title *Leizheng puji ben shi fang* 類證普濟本事方 (*Original Formulary of Classified Manifestation Types for Popular Relief*).

13   Cullen (2001, 309) claimed that Xu's format of presenting the case details did not follow the Ming's "*an*" style and "served as a mere adjunct to other forms of writing." Furth (2007b, 129) claimed that these cases showcased the "art of prescription, the preeminent medical skill that formed the rhetorical and clinical climax of case history narratives in the mature Chinese medical tradition."

14   I claim that Xu perceived this as a new means of transmitting knowledge or a new genre since he used case histories in two of his books—the *Shanghan jiushi lun* and the *Puji benshi fang*—recording over 150 medical cases in total.

as hints included within the texts, it seems that Xu wrote a trilogy of books on the topic of Cold Damage disorders in order to facilitate readers' access to this knowledge, explain and clarify Cold Damage doctrines, and show how this newly revived ancient knowledge could and should be integrated into clinical practice.

Historical Context

Chinese medicine in 1127 CE was strikingly different from Chinese medicine a mere century and a half earlier in 960 CE. A profound transformation had reshaped medical theory, practice, and training during the course of the Northern Song dynasty (960–1127 CE). For example, the number of medical books published increased dramatically, the number of medicinal materials recorded in materia medica collections more than doubled, and the ingredients, dosages, and functions of each component of the medicinal formulas on record changed. These changes and many more transformed the medical environment in which physicians practiced after the eleventh century.[15] The most important change was the increase in accessibility and availability of medical texts both new and ancient, the majority of which were published by the Song government. During the Song dynasty, for the first time in Chinese history emperors and high officials actively showed interest in medicine.[16] The Song government promoted projects to collect medical texts, to compare surviving editions and correct errors, to revise their contents, to print them, and finally to disseminate copies to the localities. The first such project of collecting and printing medical books took place from the 970s to the 990s, when the government printed mostly books concerning drugs and formulas.[17] During the 1020s and 1030s, the government launched a second project of publishing medical books, this time focusing on canonical medical works, namely, books concerning acu-moxa therapy and revised editions of two ancient texts—the *Yellow Emperor's Inner Canon* and the *Yellow Emperor's Canon of Eighty-One Problems*.[18] The government's involvement in shaping medical knowledge reached

---

15   Goldschmidt 2005, 2009.

16   Goldschmidt 2009, chaps. 1, 2, 4.

17   Two significant books resulted from this project: the *Kaibao Reign Materia Medica* (*Kaibao bencao* 開寶本草) and the *Imperial Grace Formulary* (*Taiping sheng hui fang* 太平聖惠方).

18   Classical, or canonical, medicine—a refined, cosmological, doctrine-laden, patient-centered medicine—evolved during the last two centuries BCE. It is represented by the medical canons of the Han dynasty (206 BCE–220 CE), especially the *Yellow Emperor's Inner*

a pinnacle during the 1050s and 1060s with the establishment of a specialized office designed to revise and print medical literature—the Bureau for Emending Medical Texts (Jiaozheng yishu ju 校正醫書局, in short, the Bureau). One last project of printing medical books took place during the reign of Emperor Huizong (1101–1126).

The government established the Bureau for Emending Medical Texts in reaction to a wave of epidemics that swept the empire.[19] It can be argued that this wave of epidemics may have been exaggerated due to overly diligent officials or an emperor, Renzong, who was too concerned with omens, but that is beside the point.[20] The fact of the matter is that Emperor Renzong (1010–1063) saw these epidemics as a threat to his rule and, consequently, implemented various measures to cope with them. Establishing the Bureau was not Renzong's first reaction, but it was the one with the most lasting effects.[21] The Bureau published, printed, and disseminated a total of ten books in large numbers, and it even printed some of them in small and less expensive editions during the 1080s and 1090s. These newly printed medical treatises became the most prominent and widely used texts of Chinese medicine, in the process creating a new context for medical practice. The selection of books to be included in the project was not trivial. The original list included, as expected, well-known medical books, the majority of which had already been revised and printed under imperial auspices. The final list of books to be published by the Bureau was rather different. The most noticeable difference was the inclusion of three versions of the *Treatise on Cold Damage and Miscellaneous Disorders* (*Shanghan zabing lun* 傷寒雜病論), dating to the third century CE and written by Zhang Ji 張機 (150–219, also known as Zhang Zhongjing 张仲景), who was an official-turned-physician. The editors at the Bureau included Zhang's treatise among the books they edited and printed because of its alleged importance in treating epidemics.[22] Indeed, in the preface that they wrote to the revised ver-

---

Canon (*Huangdi neijing* 黃帝內經) and the *Yellow Emperor's Canon of Eighty-One Problems* (*Huangdi bashiyi nan jing* 黃帝八十一難經). This medical genre or approach explained the working of the human body in terms of concepts derived from Warring States and Han dynasty cosmological doctrines: namely, microcosm-macrocosm, yin-yang 陰陽, and Five Phases (*wuxing* 五行).

19   Goldschmidt 2007; 2009, chap. 3.

20   Skonicki 2007.

21   Before establishing the Bureau, Emperor Renzong sent physicians to affected areas, distributed medications without charge, and ordered the compilation, printing, and distribution of two brief formularies.

22   This was Zhang's claim in the preface to his book. From the Song dynasty on, the title was shortened to *Shanghan lun* 傷寒論 (*Treatise on Cold Damage Disorders*). The Song ver-

sion, the Bureau's editors pointed out that "of all the diseases [lit. "of the one hundred diseases"], Cold Damage disorders are the most pressing."[23] Unlike the other texts that the Bureau published, the *Treatise*, although considered important, was not meticulously annotated. The Bureau's editors clarified ambiguous characters but added very little commentary regarding the contents of the text or its doctrines. It seems that the editors, including the physicians working at the Bureau, did not possess the necessary knowledge about the doctrines and practices connected with Cold Damage disorders to provide full annotation for the readers.[24]

The Bureau's publications by themselves would probably have created some change in the medical environment, but such a change would have been limited to scholarly, rather than practical, interest in medicine. Physicians or scholars with such textual tastes would have had to seek the imperial libraries in order to gain access to these books. The Song government's ambitions to act benevolently, especially in terms of spreading practical medical knowledge, were, however, much bolder: the Song government wished to educate a new generation of physicians. Therefore, it established a medical education system in 1044. By the 1070s and 1080s and also during the early decades of the twelfth century, this education system became prominent and widespread and was supplemented with a system of medical examinations mimicking the official imperial examination system, which had also undergone many changes during that time.[25] During this second phase, the curriculum of the imperial medical education system was based on the newly available knowledge and printed medical canon circulated by the Bureau.

The medical education and examination system, which served as a means of obtaining medical positions in the bureaucracy, especially during the reign of Emperor Huizong, ensured that its graduates were proficient in all the imperially published medical texts. The increased availability of these books created, in turn, a unique situation in which a growing number of physicians and officials were proficient in a set of medical treatises that espoused doctrines

---

sion of the book is titled *Song ben Shanghan lun* 宋本傷寒論 (*Song Edition of the "Treatise"*).

23   Okanishi 1969, 352.

24   The editors did not have any information since the readership of the original *Treatise on Cold Damage Disorders* was very limited, to the point that even when medical authors mentioned Cold Damage disorders, they failed to cite Zhang Zhongjing or his book. In some other cases physicians such as Sun Simiao complained that they could not obtain a complete copy of the *Treatise*. The result was that very few books on Cold Damage existed until the Song dynasty.

25   Wang 2006; Liang 2004.

and treatments that were not compatible with contemporary medical practices.[26] This was especially true regarding the three versions of the *Treatise on
Cold Damage Disorders*, since this book was not available to the great majority
of physicians from the third century up until 1065, when the government printed the official imperial versions.

As mentioned before, the first problem Song physicians had to address, and
apparently the most pressing one according to their own accounts, was the
increasing frequency of epidemics. In 1086 Han Zhihe 韓祗和 described a situation in which 70–80 percent of the population were severely affected by
Cold Damage disorders:

> Already thirty years have passed from the time of the Zhihe 至和 reign
> period [1054–1055] to the present. Disregarding the effects of the increase
> or decrease in the number of [sick people in] a given year, the number of
> people struck by Cold Damage before the summer solstice has been
> seven or eight out of ten…. Because they [contemporary physicians] did
> not dare to recklessly prescribe Zhongjing's drug treatments for Three Yin
> disorder, physicians only observed the floating pulse and fullness at the
> chest and diaphragm, and then they prescribed bringing-down [purging]
> drugs. Frequently [this type of treatment did] not save [the patient].[27]

In order to cope with this disturbing reality, physicians began to study the newly printed *Treatise*. But since this book represented third-century unrevised
and unedited medical knowledge, Song physicians had to update and integrate
the *Treatise*'s diagnostic techniques and prescriptions with contemporary clinical practices and norms. Three physicians stood out in these attempts: Han
Zhihe 韓祗和 (ca. 1030–1100), who elaborated on pulse diagnostic techniques,
which were closely tied to classical medicine; Pang Anshi 龐安時 (1042–1099),
who resolved the ambiguity in the nosology of Cold Damage disorders, their
associated symptoms, and the preferred treatment for each type of Cold Damage disorder; and Zhu Gong 朱肱 (fl. late eleventh and early twelfth centuries),
who was the first to try and integrate classical doctrines with Cold Damage
doctrines. Though concentrating on terminology and diagnosis-related assumptions, these physicians brought about a significant transition from the
earlier clinically oriented discussion.

At this point in our story we come to Xu Shuwei, who followed the above
three, and the ways in which he confronted the problems of understanding,

---

26   Wang 2006; Liang 2004.
27   *Shanghan wei zhi lun, juan* 2, 23.

promulgating, and integrating Cold Damage disorders by means of a new literary genre of medical case histories. We now have to consider the question that
Xu faced in writing his books: how to transmit medical information to posterity, especially clinical information?

Xu Shuwei's Personal History

Xu Shuwei was a Song dynasty physician from a locality named Baisha 白沙 in
Zhen Prefecture 真州 (present-day Jiangsu). He came from a poor family that
was not part of a lineage of physicians; his father served in the military. When
Xu was eleven, his father succumbed to a "seasonal epidemic" 時疫. A few
months later, a hundred days to be precise, he lost his mother to a disease as
well.[28] This traumatic loss occurring at such a young age took a great toll on
young Xu, as is evident from the preface he wrote to his formulary decades
later:

> When I was eleven years old, we continuously encountered family mis
> fortune. My father caught a seasonal epidemic 時疫, and my mother had
> a syndrome called *qizhong* 氣中 disorder.[29] Within one hundred days, I
> had lost them both. I was anguished by the thought that there was not a
> single good doctor in our village [who could help them]. I and my mother
> and then I alone waited powerless for the [inevitable] end. When I grew
> up, I painstakingly read all available formularies [I could find]. I swore
> wholeheartedly to devote my life to saving all living beings. Amid the
> murk there seems to have been something that guided me as the years
> went by. Now I am old and have already collected an extensive number of
> proven formulas. I also have come to the point of ascribing new meaning
> [to medicine].[30]

At the beginning of his formulary, where he presented his mother's disease as
a case history, Xu reiterated his frustration with the inadequate medical care
available to his family during his parents' sickness. He described her symptoms
and the treatment she received only to conclude that if the attending doctor

---

28   Zhao 2012, 5–6; Chen 1989, 1–3; Liu and Li 2006, 169–171.

29   This is a type of "being struck by wind" (*zhongfeng* 中風) disorder. This disorder arises
      from an excess of feelings of depression or anger, which causes the liver's *qi* to flow contrary to its designated path. See Li et al. 2005, 310.

30   *Puji ben shi fang*, 83; Okanishi 1969, 845–846.

had been competent, he would have realized that he had misdiagnosed her and that she in fact had a disease that could have been easily treated and cured. Xu provided the diagnosis as well as the recommended treatment for the correct disease in his case history while reiterating the incompetence of the attending doctor.[31]

The inability of local physicians to help his ailing parents and prevent their deaths, as well as the need to earn a living, motivated Xu to study medicine. He focused on Cold Damage disorders since his father's disorder fell under this general category of disorders. Besides pursuing a medical career, Xu never relinquished his dream of passing the civil service examinations. In 1132, after repeatedly failing them, he finally passed the highest level of the imperial examinations, ranked fifth no less, and became an official at the age of fifty-three. Subsequently, he was appointed to a number of official teaching and scholarly positions, including serving as a scholar at the Imperial Hanlin Academy. Consequently, he acquired the nickname Xu the Scholar 許學士. Xu was a prolific writer, authoring about ten titles; however, only four of his texts have survived to the present.[32] The renowned Qing dynasty doctor Xu Bin 徐彬 (fl. late seventeenth century) summed up Xu Shuwei's standing among those who studied Cold Damage disorders: "from antiquity, among the sages of Cold Damage only Zhang Zhongjing [stands out]. Of those who promoted and honored [Zhang] Zhongjing and interpreted [his work], singly Xu Shuwei was the best."[33]

Xu's Trilogy on Cold Damage Disorders

Xu Shuwei, like many physicians during the late eleventh and early twelfth centuries, struggled with the government's printing of the *Song Edition of the Treatise on Cold Damage Disorders* (*Song ben shanghan lun* 宋本傷寒論). The availability of this centuries-old, unadulterated medical knowledge dating to the third century CE provided a unique challenge since it did not conform to contemporary, Song dynasty medical practice. Xu and his peer physicians highly regarded this text, which had been praised and coveted by doctors for centuries while only a handful had access to it.[34] Xu praised the *Treatise* and

---

31   *Puji ben shi fang*, 92.

32   Liu and Li 2006, 169–171; *Zhizhai shulu jieti.*

33   *Zhongguo yiji kao, juan* 31; Yan et al. 1990–1994, 422; also quoted in Liu and Li 2006, 183.

34   Goldschmidt 2009, chap. 5. The best evidence for the limited accessibility of the *Treatise* before the Song dynasty can be found in the Tang dynasty physician Sun Simiao's preface to his *Essential Recipes Worth a Thousand Gold Pieces, for Urgent Need*, where he

warned his readers that "discussing Cold Damage disorders without reading [Zhang] Zhongjing's book [the *Treatise*] is like discussing Confucianism without first understanding the six canons of Confucius."[35] This statement suggests that contemporary physicians diagnosed and treated patients afflicted by Cold Damage disorders according to fixed patterns of symptoms without understanding the underlying causes according to the doctrines of the *Treatise*. During the last decades of the Northern Song, we find increasing numbers of complaints from educated doctors suggesting that the practice of treating symptoms without understanding the underlying pathology had become much more prominent. The advancement in printing leading to the accessibility of medical literature, as well as the government initiative to promote the sale of the Imperial Pharmacy's prepared prescriptions, may account for the rise of so-called physicians who were susceptible to this type of criticism.[36]

At first sight, Xu's three books do not stand out except for the fact that the third is the first collection of medical case histories compiled by a Chinese physician. In order to understand how these three books form a trilogy and why Xu constructed them this way and included the case histories in the last one, we need to take a step back and contextualize Xu's medical environment. This was a radically new environment that experienced democratization of medical knowledge in the form of increased access to printed medical books and contemporary works. Thus, knowledge that traditionally was transmitted only within family lineages or master-disciple lines became available to a much wider audience.

Xu's three books discussing Cold Damage disorders complement each other while serving different purposes and form a trilogy of books that were probably intended to be read together. Below I delineate the content and structure of each of these three books in order to show how they relate to each other and how they grew out of one another. I claim that Xu wrote these three books successively to enhance the understanding of Cold Damage disorders among his peers. To achieve this goal Xu structured the three books in a way that was intended to facilitate the transmission of both theoretical and clinical knowledge about Cold Damage disorders, knowledge he deemed indispensable yet gravely lacking among physicians. To ensure that a broad audience of readers

---

comments that "in Jiangnan [a region in South China] there are various masters who conceal Zhang Ji's essential formulary and do not transmit it." It took Sun thirty years to obtain part of the *Treatise* in 682. See *Beiji qianjin yaofang*, chaps. 9 and 10.

35   *Shanghan baizheng ge* 百證歌; Okanishi 1969, 443–444.
36   Goldschmidt 2008.

could easily comprehend his understanding of this newly rediscovered field of medicine, Xu decided to use a number of literary styles.

It seems that while writing his trilogy of books concerning Cold Damage disorders Xu struggled with two major issues. The first was how to ensure his audience's familiarity with and comprehension of the contents of the *Treatise*. The second was how to educate his audience about the intricacies of integrating the *Treatise*'s Cold Damage doctrines with contemporary clinical practice. Accordingly, Xu designed his first book to address the first issue and the latter two to address the second. In writing his first book, *One Hundred Mnemonic Verses on Cold Damage Manifestations* (*Shanghan bai zheng ge* 傷寒百證歌),[37] Xu implemented a literary tool he learned while studying for his civil service examinations, namely, setting the original content of the *Treatise* into easy-to-remember rhymes, a tool still widely used for memorizing substantial amounts of material among contemporary medical students. In the preface to his *One Hundred Mnemonic Verses on Cold Damage Manifestations*, Xu writes: "Hence I took the contents of the *Treatise* and compiled from it one hundred mnemonic poems, each delineating a manifestation type. I did this to make it easier for physicians to study and memorize it [the *Treatise*]."[38] By creating an easily memorized primer, Xu made an important contribution to the dissemination and popularization of the *Treatise*'s doctrines.

The *One Hundred Mnemonic Verses* consists of five fascicles, each discussing twenty manifestation types. The first two fascicles focus on the *Treatise*'s broader issues such as "inner" and "outer" manifestation types and manifestation related to "heat sensations" 發熱 and "Wind Strike" 中風. The other three fascicles focus on more specific manifestation types. The discussion of each manifestation type begins with rhymed verses in which each line consists of seven characters. Following each rhymed section, Xu quotes from the original text of the *Treatise* to clarify and elaborate. He also quotes from other ancient sources, from Tang dynasty books compiled by the Bureau for Emending Medical Texts, and from books by contemporary Song dynasty physicians.

In his second book Xu presents his personal understanding of Cold Damage doctrines and their clinical application. The *Subtleties of Cold Damage Revealed* (*Shanghan fa wei lun* 傷寒發微論) consists of two fascicles presenting

---

37   "Manifestation types" (*zheng* 證) are classifications of symptoms into general categories (or the abstract schematic characterizations of the patient's condition) that determine the treatment strategies. "Manifestation type," though similar, is not identical in meaning to "syndrome." The former is a more flexible classification than the latter, since it accords with the perception that medical disorders are dynamic processes rather than static states. For further discussion, see Sivin 1987, 106–111; Farquhar 1994, 147–174.

38   *Shanghan bai zheng ge* 百證歌; Okanishi 1969, 443–444.

twenty-two discussions (*lun* 論). It seems that Xu chose the discussion topics to represent the most important yet difficult-to-understand clinical issues in the *Treatise*. Following each of these discussions, Xu adds his own observations and conclusions regarding the topic, and here we find the first merging of, and sometimes conflict between, the classical doctrines in the *Treatise* and contemporary accumulated medical knowledge. The *Subtleties of Cold Damage Revealed* is rather brief and seems to be incomplete. It is certainly not as comprehensive as the first or the third book he authored; perhaps while writing this book Xu realized its limitations in transmitting his clinical knowledge about practical application of Cold Damage doctrines and did not complete it. It is important to note that Xu copied almost verbatim a few of the twenty-two discussions from this book into his third.

The first discussion in the *Subtleties* enumerates seventy-two manifestation types of Cold Damage, each with a brief one-line description. Starting with the second discussion, Xu explains specific manifestation types of Cold Damage disorders, focusing on their clinical aspects, such as pulse diagnosis, general diagnosis, transmitted formulas, and important issues related to prescribing medications. For each of the manifestation types, Xu quotes from the relevant section of the *Treatise* and then provides annotations, explanations, and additional information designed to enhance the reader's understanding. In some of these discussions he points out important themes in the disorder's pathology, physiology, or both, while in others he provides instructions on which drug to use, when and how to use it, and even how to prepare it. In yet other cases he discusses the prognosis of the condition in a very succinct manner. It seems to me that Xu realized the limits of existing methods of transmission, which led him to focus on case histories in his third book.

Xu's most interesting book is the *Ninety Discussions on Cold Damage Disorders* (*Shanghan jiushi lun* 傷寒九十論). In this book Xu collected ninety of his own medical case histories spanning a period of a few decades. Of Xu's three books concerning Cold Damage disorders, this one has the least documented history. All three of Xu's Cold Damage books were printed during the Qiandao 乾道 reign period of the Southern Song dynasty (1165–1173). Unlike the other two books, the *Ninety Discussions* quickly fell out of circulation, to the point of being considered lost. A printed version of the book resurfaced during the Qing dynasty in the hands of an avid book collector named Zhang Jinwu 張金吾 (1787–1829).[39] Nevertheless, case histories from Xu's *Ninety Discussions* were quoted abundantly, often verbatim, in various medical books and Ming dynas-

---

39   Liu and Li 2006, 170–171; Chen 1989, 2–4. The surviving printed copy we have today is dated to 1853 (咸豐三年) and is part of the *Linlang mishi congshu* 琳琅秘室叢書 (vol. 11).

ty collections of case histories (*yi'an* 醫案), including in the renowned *Cases of Famous Physicians Arranged by Category* (*Mingyi lei'an* 名醫類案).[40] Xu's book has no preface or introduction to elaborate on the author's goals or intentions; there is also no information regarding the selection method of its content. With no evidence to rely on, we can only assume that Xu himself chose the cases in the book, perhaps indicating that these were the best possible examples of the knowledge he wanted to transmit to his readers.

Each of the cases presents a clinical scene that represents important points of the *Treatise*. Several of the cases in the *Ninety Discussions on Cold Damage Disorders* also appear almost verbatim in Xu's *Original Formulary for Popular Relief*, indicating their importance. The *Ninety Discussions* serves as the third and final layer of Xu's project of transmitting knowledge about Cold Damage disorders. In this layer he explains how he chooses among Cold Damage manifestation types for specific cases and then adds a theoretical discussion explaining his actions.

Xu's Cases

Xu's third book deserves further discussion since it is the most innovative of the three. Xu's collection of case histories stands starkly alone, as none of his peers and successors imitated his example and produced similar collections of case histories. Only during the Ming dynasty, some 250 years later, did the literary genre of medical case histories become popular. In order to understand Xu's motivation for authoring such an innovative book, we need to discuss the cases themselves and see what themes tie them together. It seems that Xu chose to utilize this genre in order to highlight various mundane medical issues.

All the cases in Xu's *Ninety Discussions* follow a similar general structure. Nevertheless, many of the case histories also elaborate further on the issues discussed in the specific case. Each of the cases begins with some personal details about the patient, such as name, locale, social status, and sometime even the patient's ranks or personal relationship to Xu. The duration of the disease, its major symptoms, and its changes or development over time are given next. The list of symptoms that follows is rather detailed, especially in comparison to other medical records surviving from the Tang and Song dynasties. The most important detail Xu provides is the pulse that he has taken at the patient's wrists. In some cases, Xu delineates the symptoms in a specific order

---

40   *Mingyi lei'an*, 23, 25, 27, 51, 65–66, 184, 185, 188, 244, 318, 343–344.

to single out one symptom that requires closer attention by the physician since the diagnosis hinges on it. In some of the cases, Xu documents the treatment that other doctors prescribed to the patient in order to point out its problems and how it was the result of a misdiagnosis. Once Xu has stated the diagnosis of the patient's disorder, he lists the corresponding treatment. In the majority of the cases, Xu applies a formula taken from Zhang Zhongjing's *Treatise* as a treatment. However, in at least three cases, Xu specifically states that the *Treatise* does not record a treatment for the condition but that he has devised a treatment from his own clinical experience.[41] It seems that as much as he revered the *Treatise*, his own accumulated clinical experience was just as important. Following the treatment, Xu often provides a short quotation from the *Treatise* and then a description of the effects of the treatment on the patient. In some of the cases, Xu expands on the clinical scene and records conversations he had with members of the patient's family or with a physician present at the scene. In these dialogues Xu answers direct questions posed to him regarding his diagnosis, treatment, and the sources of his knowledge.

The majority of Xu's case records do not end after his report of the outcome of the patient's disorder but include a second part titled "discussion." This part of the case record consists of a theoretical discussion concerning the origin of the symptoms, the rationale behind the diagnosis of the manifestation type, or an explanation of the treatment. This discussion is unique to Xu's case histories, since here Xu details how his clinical case record draws from the doctrines and practices of the ancient medical books reprinted during the Northern Song dynasty. In some of the cases, the discussion is almost a verbatim repetition of sections from Xu's second book, *Subtleties of Cold Damage Revealed*. This fact supports the supposition that Xu never completed the second book and regarded it as a failed attempt to transmit knowledge. Once Xu came up with the idea to employ case histories as a means to facilitate the transmission of clinical knowledge, he readily incorporated these earlier discussions into the new format.

Since cases are at the heart of my essay, I will now provide translations of a few of Xu's cases, followed by a brief delineation of the main points they discuss. These cases represent the types of theoretical and practical issues Xu faced when treating patients with Cold Damage disorders. Xu, by presenting these cases, stresses to the reader issues such as differential diagnosis, differentiation between symptoms, and the strategy for choosing treatments in the clinical context. Additionally, he also provides the reader with the social and professional context in which he practiced. Xu's cases also include many

---

41   For example, see cases 4, 9, and 10.

rhetorical tools to enhance the transmission of the clinical information to the reader. The majority of the cases include brief dialogues and even confrontations between Xu and other physicians or the patient's family members. Xu extensively quotes medical sources, including but not solely the *Treatise*.

Case 1: Clarifying the Debate concerning the Use of Chinese Herbaceous Peony Root in the Cassia Twig Decoction Manifestation Type 辯桂枝湯用芍藥證

During the spring of the Gengxu year [1130], Mr. Ma Hengdao became sick.[42] He experienced hot sensations,[43] headache, noisy nose,[44] nausea, spontaneous sweating, and aversion to wind.[45] All these symptoms pointed to a Cassia Twig manifestation type.[46] During this time, mounted bandits[47] have been raiding the city of Yizhen[48] for three days straight. [Since] drug sellers in the city markets had no peony root for sale [to be included in the decoction for this manifestation type], I went to my herb garden, picked a peony [Chinese herbaceous peony], and completed the prescription. One doctor said, "This is red peony root. How can you use it [as an ingredient in this prescription]?" I said, "This is exactly what [the patient] should consume [as part of the decoction]." The patient had two sips from the decoction, perspired a little, and [the disorder] was resolved.

Discussion: As for Zhongjing's[49] Cassia Twig adding and reducing method, it is recorded in nineteen [of the *Treatise*'s] manifestation types, but

---

42   During the years following the Jurchen conquest of the Northern Song dynasty, the regions north and south of the lower Yangzi River were often the setting for repeated military confrontations between the troops of the Southern Song and the Jurchen Jin dynasty. Xu Shuwei resided in Zhen Prefecture 真州 (present-day Jiangsu), which is located in this area.

43   The phrase *fa re* 發熱 refers both to fever and to having heat sensations that may or may not coincide with the Western understanding of "fever." I prefer to translate *fa re* 發熱 as "hot sensations" since this conveys a much broader sense of the symptom and is probably closer to the full scope of the term as perceived by physicians during the Song dynasty.

44   "Noisy nose" (*bi ming* 鼻鳴) refers to coarse breathing like that caused by a stuffy nose.

45   "Aversion to wind" (*efeng* 惡風) refers to when the patient feels unusual discomfort when exposed to wind.

46   For a discussion of Cassia Twig manifestation types in the *Treatise*, see Mitchell, Ye, and Wiseman 1999, 59–75.

47   The characters *zeima* 賊馬 (robbers and horses) often referred to Jurchen soldiers as well during the Song dynasty.

48   Yizhen was a township in Zhen Prefecture 真州 (present-day Jiangsu).

49   This is a shorthand reference to Zhang Zhongjing, the author of the *Treatise on Cold Damage and Miscellaneous Disorders*.

when discussing peony root, the *Imperial Grace Formulary*[50] records all as red peony root. In the book titled *Sun Shang's Drugs and Formulas* 孫尚藥方,[51] however, all references are to white peony root. The *Imperial Grace Formulary* was collected and compiled by Wang Huaiyin during the reign of Song Taizong [976–997]. Sun Zhao was a Master Physician[52] [during the Northern Song dynasty] and should not have taken the completely opposite interpretation [of which peony to use]. Certainly, the red peony root is used to drain, whereas the white peony root is used to supplement. I once raised this difficult issue with a number of famous physicians, all of whom were astounded and baffled by it.

My humble notes: The *Divine Husbandman's Materia Medica* states that peony root controls evil *qi* that is causing pain in the abdomen, drains the urine, clears and smoothes the blood vessels, and drains the urinary bladder, the large intestine, and the small intestine tracts. [It also cures] chills and heat sensations due to unseasonable weather.[53] [Given this and the above information,] then this is all [treated] by red peony root. Furthermore, [the *Treatise*'s] ninth Cassia Twig manifestation type states: "In cases of minor cold, discard the red peony root."[54] This is due to the fear of the coldness trait of this drug. Only one manifestation type—that of Peony Root and Licorice Decoction—mentions white peony root, with the symptom of the patient's two legs having difficulty flexing due to coldness in the blood. Therefore, one has to supplement with white peony root, [but] this condition is not due to the effects of the season [it is caused by an internal problem, not external effects]. The *Suwen* volume of the *Inner Canon* states: "As for rough [pulse], it is due to excess yang *qi*. When there is excess yang *qi*, this causes the body to be hot and without sweat. When the yin *qi* is in excess, it causes the body to be cold and to sweat a lot. In Cold Damage [disorders] the pulse is rough, the body is hot, and there is no sweat. Thus, it means that evil *qi* attacked the yin *qi*, and consequently the yang *qi* is in excess. There is only herba ephedra to

---

50   The *Imperial Grace Formulary of the Great Peace and Prosperity Reign Period* (*Taiping sheng hui fang* 太平聖惠方) was the first grand formulary published during the Song dynasty. Its author was Wang Huaiyin 王懷隱 (fl. 978–992), and it appeared in 992.

51   This refers to a book written by Sun Yonghe 孙用和 (fl. mid-eleventh century, also known as Sun Zhao 孫兆 and Sun Shang 孫尚), who was a famous scholar-physician.

52   Hucker 1985, 269.

53   This sentence is an incomplete quotation from the Peony section of the *Divine Husbandman's Materia Medica* (*Shennong bencao jing* 神農本草經), *juan* 8, 16.

54   This is a direct quotation from the *Treatise*; see Mitchell, Ye, and Wiseman 1999, 87; Yu et al. 1997, 38.

be used to disperse [this condition]." When attacked by wind, the pulse is slippery, there is profuse sweating, and the body is cold. Thus, it means that the evil *qi* attacked the yang. Therefore, the yin *qi* is in excess. Only red peony root can be used to eliminate its evil yin. In the case of the current patient then, the choice of using red peony root to prepare the Cassia Twig Decoction is clear. One may consult [my book] *One Hundred Mnemonic Verses on Cold Damage Manifestations.*[55]

馬亨道，庚戌春病。發熱，頭疼，鼻鳴，惡心，自汗，惡風，宛然桂枝證也。時賊馬破儀真三日矣，市無芍藥，自指[詣][56]圃園，采芍藥以利劑。一醫曰：此赤芍藥耳，安可用也？予曰：此正當用，再啜而微汗解。

論曰：仲景桂枝加減法，十有九證，但雲芍藥，《聖惠方》皆稱赤芍藥，《孫尚藥方》皆曰白芍藥。《聖惠方》，太宗朝翰林王懷隱編集，孫兆為國朝醫師，不應如此背戾，然赤者利，白者補。予嘗以此難名醫，皆愕然失措。

謹案：《神農本草》稱，芍藥主邪氣腹痛，利小便，通順血脈，利膀胱大小腸，時行寒熱，則全是赤芍藥也。又桂枝第九證雲：微寒者，去赤芍藥。蓋懼芍藥之寒也。惟芍藥甘草湯一證雲白芍藥，謂其兩脛拘急，血寒也。故用白芍藥以補，非此時也。《素問》雲：澀者陽氣有余也。陽氣有余為身熱無汗，陰氣有余為多汗身寒。傷寒脈澀，身熱無汗，蓋邪中陰氣，故陽有余，非麻黃不能發散。中風脈滑，多汗身寒，蓋邪中陽，故陰有余，非赤芍藥不能刮[劫]其陰邪。然則桂枝用芍藥赤者明矣。當參《百證歌》。

This case history focuses on an issue that to the lay observer may seem innocuous and maybe not even important but that in reality represents one of the major problems physicians had to cope with during the Song dynasty. The issue is whether to include red or white peony root in prescriptions, in general, and in formulas designed to treat Cold Damage disorders, in particular. This

---

55   Here Xu refers to his book *One Hundred Mnemonic Verses on Cold Damage Manifestations* (*Shanghan bai zheng ge* 傷寒百證歌) in a shorthand form: *Bai zheng ge* 百證歌.

56   These two characters differ in different versions of the book. In the *Zhongguo yixue dacheng* version (volume 3, p. 31) the character *yi* 詣 (with a speech radical) appears. The character *zhi* 指 (with a hand radical) appears in the *Congshu jicheng* edition, in the *Xuxiu siku quanshu*, and in the modern reproductions.

controversy came about because of the government-sponsored printing of ancient medical books, including the *Treatise on Cold Damage and Miscellaneous Disorders*, whose contents did not align with advancing medical practice. The *Treatise* in many places mentions only peony root; however, over the centuries physicians came to use two types of peony, white and red. Xu uses the case to highlight this discrepancy between ancient and contemporary clinical knowledge by discussing the different effects of the two drugs. He presents the disagreement in contemporary medical literature regarding which one is correct. Finally, he claims that the correct peony for the case at hand is the red one and provides references to two additional sources to support his position. Altogether Xu refers to five different texts in discussing this topic. Lastly, reading this case we learn that during the Song dynasty patients obtained the drugs to make their medications both in the markets and from the private gardens of their physicians.

Case 2: Manifestation Type [Requiring Treatment with] Prepared Aconite Root Added to Cassia Twig Decoction 桂枝加附子湯證

There was a literatus surnamed Li. He contracted a Taiyang[57] [disorder]. Because of a [medical] treatment inducing sweating, he did not stop perspiring [from that point in time on].[58] He also experienced aversion to wind and difficulties in urinating, and lastly, his leg had spasms and was flexed without the ability to stretch. I palpated his pulse and found it to be floating and large. Floating pulse indicates wind pathogen and large pulse indicates deficiency. This was the seventh manifestation type for Cassia Twig Decoction. Zhongjing said, "In disorders of the Taiyang [circulation tract], the patient begins sweating, and he leaks water without stop. This person has aversion to wind, it is difficult for him to urinate, and his four limbs are lightly tensed, [resulting] in difficulty in bending and stretching them. In these cases add aconite to the Cassia Twig [Decoction]."[59] After I administered to him three doses [of the prescription], the sweating stopped. Next, I gave the patient Peony and Liquorice Decoction. Consequently, the patient was able to stretch his legs. After several days, the patient was cured.

---

57 This is a shorthand reference to the manifestation type "Taiyang struck by wind" (*taiyang zhong feng* 太陽中風).

58 This refers to a situation in which a doctor applies a sweating technique but the patient continues to sweat even after the treatment's effects end.

59 This is a direct quotation from the *Treatise*; see Mitchell, Ye, and Wiseman 1999, 83–84; Yu et al. 1997, 38.

Discussion: Zhongjing's sixteenth manifestation type [of Cassia Twig] states: "In [cases of] Cold Damage disorders [when] the pulse is floating, there is spontaneous sweating, urination is frequent, the heart is irritated, there is a mild aversion to cold, and the foot is tense and has spasms, it is a mistake to treat [this condition] by administering Cassia Twig Decoction to attack the exterior. If [the patient] consumes this [decoction], then there will be reversal; namely, his larynx will be dry, and he will be vexed and agitated and will vomit. These symptoms are treatable with Licorice Root and Dried Ginger Decoction. If the reversal is cured and the feet become warm, then make Peony and Licorice Decoction and offer it to the patient, and subsequently [his or her] feet will then [be able to] stretch. If the stomach's *qi* is disharmonious and there is delirious speech, administer to the patient a little Adjust the Stomach and Hold the Qi Decoction."[60] In fact, [if the case at hand is] the seventh manifestation type, then inducing sweating will cause a leakage without stop and difficulty urinating. [If the case at hand is the] sixteenth manifestation type, then there will be spontaneous sweating and frequent urination. Therefore, [Zhang] Zhongjing, in discussing manifestation types and symptoms, [listed] one after another small variation, conveniently changing strategies in order to cure [the disorder]. Therefore, with regard to this decoction, one must be very cautious.

有一李姓士人，得太陽，因汗後汗不止，惡風，小便澀，足攣曲而不伸。予診其脈，浮而大，浮為風，大為虛，此證桂枝湯第七證也。仲景雲：太陽病，發汗，遂漏不止，其人惡風，小便難，四肢微急，難以屈伸者，桂枝加附子。三投而汗止，再投以芍藥甘草，而足得伸。數日愈。

論曰：仲景第十六證雲：『傷寒，脈浮，自汗出，小便數，心煩，微惡寒，腳攣急，反與桂枝湯以攻其表，此誤也。得之便厥，咽中幹，煩躁吐逆者，作甘草幹姜湯。若厥愈足溫者，更作芍藥甘草湯與之，其腳即伸。若胃氣不和，譫語者，少與調胃承氣湯。』蓋第七證則為發汗漏不止，小便難，第十六證則為自汗，小便數。故仲景於證候，紛紛小變異，便變法以治之，故於湯不可不謹。

---

60   This is a direct quotation from the *Treatise*; see Mitchell, Ye, and Wiseman 1999, 187–188; Yu et al. 1997, 39.

In the second case, Xu Shuwei brings to the forefront the issue of implementing canonical textual knowledge within the clinical realm. The *Treatise* discusses and classifies various Cold Damage manifestation types that are named after the appropriate treatment formula for each. A nonclinician may mistakenly think that the symptoms patients manifest are just as easily differentiated. Xu shows in this case that differentiating between similar disorders of the Cassia Twig manifestation type is far from obvious. In both manifestation types discussed in the case, the symptoms are similar except for one or two symptoms upon which differentiating the etiology hinges, thus leading to different treatment strategies. This case presents the reader with the minute distinctions necessary to diagnose correctly two similar but different Cold Damage syndromes.

Case 3: Manifestation Type [Requiring Treatment with] *Magnolia officinalis* and Apricot Added to Cassia Twig Decoction 桂枝加濃樸杏子湯證61

On the first month of the *wushen* year [1128 CE], a military official in the city of Yizhen became a prisoner of the Jurchen invaders.62 For a number of days he was held captive and was tied [in the storage space] beneath the deck in a large ship where he could not stretch. After being a captive like this for several days, he managed to escape. [Following his escape] he ate his fill, and he disrobed and brushed off fleas from his body; he was pleased with himself. Consequently, the next day, he was afflicted with a Cold Damage disorder. A certain physician thought that since he had overeaten [after escaping his imprisonment], he became sick. Accordingly, he purged him [to expel the excess]. Another doctor thought that since he disrobed, the patient was hit by evil [*qi*]. Consequently, this doctor applied sweating treatment to him [to expel the evil *qi*]. [This patient received] a number of miscellaneous treatments over several days. Gradually, he became confused and sleepy. He had upper panting and high breathing.63 The doctors who treated him were confused and scared, not knowing what caused this disorder. I diagnosed him and said, "[This is a]

---

61   This case history also appears in *Puji ben shi fang, juan* 8, p. 142.

62   In an almost identical case recorded in *Puji ben shi fang*, 142, we have the phrase "the invaders held captive" (*kousuozhi* 寇所执) instead of the name Zhang Yu 張遇. Therefore, I conclude that Zhang Yu serves as a general reference to the leader of the mounted army of the Jurchen invaders or a band of bandits. Furthermore, this is a general reference to a mounted army, probably the Jurchens.

63   "High breathing" (*xi gao* 息高) is a serious breathing difficulty in which there is severe shortness of breath and the mouth does not open completely. See Li et al. 2005, 1441.

Taiyang disorder. I need to purge it. Since the exterior is not resolved, the patient experiences slight panting. [Zhang] Zhongjing's method is to prescribe a Cassia Twig with *Magnolia officinalis* and Apricot Decoction." A doctor contended, saying, "Some [doctors], over the course of their whole lives [or careers], have never used the Cassia Twig [Decoction]. Moreover, this medication is hot [in quality]. How can it cure panting?" I said, "This is not something you know." After I administered one dose [of the decoction], the panting subsided. Upon administering the second dose, much sweat poured out. Not long afterward, the patient's body was cooler and the vessels were already harmonized. The other doctor said, "I do not know of Zhongjing's methods, nor did I realize that they are as divine as this." I said, "[Knowing] Zhongjing's methods, how could it have deceived and confused later generations? People simply do not study [this topic]; therefore, they have no way to comprehend it."

戊申正月，有一武弁在儀真為張遇所虜，日夕置於舟艎板下，不勝跧[=蜷]伏。後數日得脫，因飽食解衣捫虱以自快，次日遂作傷寒。醫者以因飽食傷而下之，一醫以解衣中邪而汗之。雜治數日，漸覺昏困，上喘息高。醫者愴惶，罔知所指。予診之曰：太陽病下之，表未解，微喘者，桂枝加濃樸杏子湯，此仲景法也。醫者爭曰：某平生不曾用桂枝，況此藥熱，安可愈喘？予曰：非汝所知也，一投而喘定，再投而漐漐汗出。至晚身涼而脈已和矣。醫者曰：予不知仲景之法，其神如此。予曰：[知]仲景之法，豈誑惑後世也哉！人自寡學，無以發明耳。

In this case Xu is tackling the task of differential diagnosis, not from the canonically based manifestation types, as delineated in the previous case, but rather from the perspective of the patient's symptoms. Xu utilizes this example to stress to the reader the importance of the fine observation skills essential in diagnosing Cold Damage disorders. The need for clear distinctions between symptoms, of course, is not unique to Cold Damage disorders, but this case provides us with a glimpse into the thought process of a Song dynasty physician and how he perceived the patient as a whole, on the one hand, and how he differentiated slight variations in symptoms to reach the correct diagnosis and treatment, on the other. In order to make his presentation more engaging, Xu frames it in a brief dialogue between himself and another doctor discussing the issues in the diagnosis. In the dialogue, the other doctor shows ignorance concerning Cold Damage disorders and their treatment. This is a recurring theme in Xu's writing that is intended to emphasize that his contemporaries lacked the necessary familiarity with the contents of the *Treatise on Cold Damage Disorders.*

Choosing Case Records as a Literary Genre

It has been suggested that spatial transmission or migration of scientific knowledge from one culture or geographic locality to another occurs in three stages: a scientist or community of scientists becomes aware of a theory or scientific technique; the new idea arouses interest and is judged to be significant; the new idea is adopted by the community.[64] This model of transmission, however, is not suited to the case at hand, since we are faced with temporal, rather than spatial, transmission: the reappearance of indigenous ancient knowledge, often in a corrupted state or unclear archaic language yet with a priori great prestige. Therefore, the need arises to better understand the text and then assimilate and integrate it into existing practices considered to be of similar descent or even direct descendants of that ancient knowledge itself. Here the process of transmission often involves a stage between that in which interest is expressed and before that in which the "new" knowledge is adopted by the community. This intermediate stage involves copying the texts, correcting errors, annotating the original texts, explaining difficult sections, or even cross-referencing the transmitted texts with existing, widely circulating texts. This stage, during the Song dynasty, was predominantly conducted and sponsored by the imperial government. The next stage involved the promulgation of the newly available texts and the assimilation process within the rank and file of doctors. This final stage is more problematic, especially when the newly available texts are circulated in their original, archaic language. In this situation, scholars or physicians first needed to rewrite the archaic knowledge in a more accessible form, using contemporary vocabulary to explain the ancient doctrines, and then, in the case of medicine, they needed to provide clinical examples. The Song government's printing of the *Treatise on Cold Damage Disorders* posed exactly such a challenge to contemporary practicing physicians, since it was incompatible with existing medical practices. Furthermore, the new bureaucratic intervention that took the form of printing medical books and establishing an imperial medical education and examination system changed the context in which physicians functioned. These changes require historians to reevaluate the common historical perception of linear transmission of knowledge or its geographical migration.

---

64   Dolby 1977, 1.

The changing environment of the Song dynasty altered the means of transmitting medical knowledge. Prior to the Song, medical knowledge was passed down in family lineages or along master-disciple lines. With the advancements in print technology and the government projects for printing medical books, physicians were exposed to new types of medical knowledge that created a crisis since it was not in line with existing practices. Furthermore, the possibility of printing books and the existence of an imperial medical education system opened new avenues for transmitting knowledge but also challenged physicians to find the best way to do so.

Xu Shuwei exemplifies the dilemma many Song dynasty physicians faced. On the one hand, the literature made newly available, especially the *Treatise*, did not conform to their existing medical knowledge or contemporary practice. On the other hand, these physicians could not ignore these works since the Song government sanctioned them as *the medical canon* and included them in the official syllabus taught at the medical schools, making them the basis of the imperial medical examinations. Xu and his peers had to integrate and reconcile this newly available ancient knowledge with their own clinically proven medical knowledge. Doing this was an innovative project since they had very limited additional literature to consult besides the ancient works themselves. Moreover, given Xu's personal biography and the fact that the Song government gave high priority to dealing with epidemics, Xu had incentives to find ways to integrate and promulgate this new knowledge about Cold Damage disorders.

Xu designed his trilogy of books to teach the doctrines of Cold Damage and how to apply them in practice. In the first book, Xu used a method he probably acquired during the long years in which he prepared for the imperial examinations: structuring the contents of the *Treatise* in rhyming mnemonic verses to facilitate memorization. Once the reader had learned the theoretical knowledge, the next stage according to Xu was to integrate the various facets of the theory of Cold Damage disorders into contemporary theoretical and clinical knowledge by cross-referencing them. Based on the incomplete form of Xu's second book, it seems that he soon realized that this type of presentation was insufficient for transmitting the new integrated knowledge. He then turned to a different manner of imparting his clinical knowledge along with its theoretical basis. In this third book, Xu used an innovative literary genre—the medical case history—combining it with a detailed doctrinal discussion to ensure, at least in his mind, that his readers would be able to comprehend and apply this method.

Xu expressed his high esteem of both medicine and doctors in the preface to his formulary: "The physician's Way [Dao] is great. He can nourish life, preserve

the body, extend years of life. In sum, he can benefit the world."[65] Xu thought
that in order to practice the "Way" of medicine, a physician had to thoroughly
know its doctrines and comprehensively understand its practice; this, however, was where he felt contemporary physicians were lacking. For example, in
case 3 above, Xu presents a patient whom several doctors diagnosed and treated, each suggesting a different treatment strategy but only worsening the patient's condition, leading to the patient's development of a panting symptom.
It was then that Xu clinically intervened with his diagnosis and prescribed Cassia Twig Decoction. Next we find a telling dialogue between Xu and another
physician who contested Xu's diagnosis, saying, "Some [doctors], over the
course of their whole lives [or careers], have never used the Cassia Twig [De-
coction]. Moreover, this medication is hot [in quality]. How can it cure panting?" Xu then replies, stating that contemporary physicians are not aware of
this treatment. Once Xu reports that the patient recovered from the disease,
the other doctor is quoted as saying, "I do not know of Zhongjing's methods,
nor did I realize that they are as divine as this." Xu then replies, claiming that
the problem is not misunderstanding of Cold Damage doctrines but that
"people simply do not study [this topic]; therefore, they have no way to comprehend it."

It is clear from this case that Xu felt that medical knowledge, especially clinical knowledge related to the *Treatise*, was not readily available. Although the
Song dynasty, following its defeat in 1127, retreated to southern China, where
seasonal epidemics and Cold Damage disorders were much more common,
contemporary physicians were not familiar with the *Treatise*'s contents or with
its clinical application. Xu must have concluded that cases histories were the
best literary means to transmit his medical knowledge to his contemporaries
and to posterity.

The clinical scenes depicted in Xu's cases have a different flavor from other
records of clinical interactions recorded before and during the Song dynasty. In
a number of them, Xu describes discussions and even arguments between
himself and other doctors or his patients. This type of interaction is not unique
to Xu's case histories and can be found elsewhere, where the "other" doctor is
often scorned as incompetent or vulgar. This was a well-established manner of
ensuring that readers understood the authoring physician's superior clinical
skill. In Xu's cases we see a different approach. Although Xu often disagreed
with the diagnosis of doctors who treated patients before him, he never called
these doctors mediocre, quacks, or charlatans (*yongyi* 庸醫). Instead, he often
mentioned their ignorance of a specific type of knowledge—the doctrines of

---

65   *Puji ben shi fang*, 83; Okanishi 1969, 845–846.

Cold Damage disorders. Consider the following examples of Xu's remarks on such ignorance:

> This is [called] the invasion of heat to the blood chamber. Those who practice medicine at the present do not know this.[66]
>
> If one prescribes Cassia Twig [Decoction, *guizhi* 桂枝], then it is to treat Wind Strike. Ephedra [Decoction, *mahuang* 麻黃], in turn, cures Cold Damage. Major Blue-Green Dragon [Decoction, *qinglong* 青龍] cures wind stroke due to cold pulse and injury by cold [pathogen] due to wind pulse. Everybody can recount these three [conditions]. But they do not know how to apply drugs that take into account the subtleties of these manifestation types. Therefore, contemporary doctors do not like using these formulas. There is no one [in particular] to blame [for this].[67]
>
> [Additionally,] the fact that both yin and yang [pulses] are tight makes these symptoms indeed perplexing. If one is not well versed in the formulas and methods of [Zhang] Zhongjing, how can he cure at all? I said, "When the pulse at both the positions of the *chi* and the *cun* is tight, this indicates that cold evil has prevailed." Zhongjing said, "When yin and yang [pulses] are both tight, the [treatment] method should be clearing. The evil attacks at the upper burner."[68]

These examples provide us with some insight concerning Xu's intentions in recording case histories. He did not aim to undermine or discredit his peers; rather, he wanted to educate them about what they did not know and what he considered essential medical knowledge for clinical practice. Xu was especially interested in Cold Damage disorders, probably due to the personal loss he suffered in his youth. Xu claimed that one of the reasons that prevailing medical practice harmed patients was that physicians either did not have access to the *Treatise* or they did not understand it. His goal was to integrate available medical literature and to explain the doctrines and treatment techniques of the *Treatise*, or in his own words: "I once talked about Zhang Zhongjing's *Treatise*.... One must use ancient and modern prescription books in order to discover and to manifest Zhongjing's immeasurable meaning."[69] Xu also knew that Cold Damage disorders and the doctrines of the *Treatise*, apart from being unavailable and unused for centuries, were also not comprehensible to

---

66   *Shanghan jiushi lun*, case 16.
67   *Shanghan jiushi lun*, case 30.
68   *Shanghan jiushi lun*, case 15.
69   *Shanghan jiushi lun*, case 84.

contemporary physicians. Although by Xu's time the reprinted *Treatise* was available and accessible, the text remained incomprehensible to the majority of contemporary physicians because the editors of the Bureau for Emending Medical Texts, as explained earlier, did not annotate it. Xu, who was also a scholar-official, had the linguistic and literary skills necessary to read and comprehend the centuries-old *Treatise*.

Concluding Remarks

From a modern prospective, Xu constructed his trilogy of books on Cold Damage disorders in an efficient and logical way for transmitting medical knowledge. In 1778 a Qing dynasty physician named Yu Zhencuan 俞震篡 also thought that Xu's work was an effective tool: "Zhongjing's *Treatise on Cold Damage Disorders* is like the Confucian canons of the *Great Learning* and the *Doctrine of the Mean*. Its language is archaic but its theoretical content is profound. From the Jin dynasty [266–316] to the present, among those proficient in applying the *Treatise*'s [knowledge], Xu Shuwei stands above all. He recorded a few dozen medical case histories and expounded them all. He did so to provide future generations with a model [to work with]."[70] However, contemporary Song dynasty and Jin dynasty (1127–1234) physicians and scholars generally disregarded Xu's books and seldom quoted them in their own works. Only a few centuries later, during the Ming, physicians copied Xu's cases into their own collections of medical case histories and his knowledge was retransmitted.

At this juncture we have no way of knowing why Xu's trilogy of books and his innovative method of transmitting medical knowledge were such failures during his own time and immediately afterward. But we may speculate that Xu's innovations were simply too far ahead of their time and that he wrote in a manner that his peers could not understand and thus failed in his goal of promoting the transmission of medical knowledge.

References

Alvarez, Millan C. 1999. "Graeco-Roman Case Histories and Their Influence on Medieval Islamic Clinical Accounts," *Social History of Medicine* 12, 1: 19–43.

—— 2010. "The Case History in Medieval Islamic Medical Literature: Tajārib and Mujarrabāt as Source," *Medical History* 54, 2: 195–214.

---

70   *Gujin yi'an an, juan* 1, 7.

Beiji qianjin yaofang 備急千金要方 [Essential recipes worth a thousand gold pieces, for urgent need]. Compiled by Sun Simiao 孫思邈, ca. 650–659. Reprint, Beijing: Huaxia chubanshi, 1993.

Chen Kezheng 陳克正 1989. *Songdai mingyi Xu Shuwei* 宋代名醫許叔微 [The famous Song physician Xu Shuwei]. Beijing: Zhongguo kexue jishu chubanshe.

Cullen, Christopher 2001. "*Yi'an* 醫案 (Case Statements): The Origins of a Genre of Chinese Medical Literature," in Elizabeth Hsu, ed., *Innovation in Chinese Medicine*. Cambridge: Cambridge University Press, 297–323.

DeWoskin, Kenneth J., trans. 1983. *Doctors, Diviners, and Magicians of Ancient China: Biographies of Fang-shih*. New York: Columbia University Press.

Dolby, R. G. A. 1977. "The Transmission of Science," *History of Science* 15: 1–43.

Farquhar, Judith 1994. *Knowing Practice: The Clinical Encounters of Chinese Medicine*. Boulder, CO: Westview Press.

Furth, Charlotte 2007a. "Introduction: Thinking with Cases," in Charlotte Furth, Judith T. Zeitlin, and Hsiung Ping-chen, eds., *Thinking with Cases: Specialist Knowledge in Chinese Cultural History*. Honolulu: University of Hawai'i Press, 1–27.

———— 2007b. "Producing Medical Knowledge through Cases: History, Evidence, and Action," in Charlotte Furth, Judith T. Zeitlin, and Hsiung Ping-chen, eds., *Thinking with Cases: Specialist Knowledge in Chinese Cultural History*. Honolulu: University of Hawai'i Press, 125–151.

Goldschmidt, Asaf 2005. "The Song Discontinuity: Rapid Innovation in Northern Song Dynasty Medicine," *Asian Medicine—Tradition and Modernity* 1, 1: 53–90.

———— 2007. "Epidemics and Medicine during the Northern Song Dynasty: The Revival of Cold Damage Disorders (*Shang han* 傷寒)," *T'oung Pao* 93, 1: 53–109.

———— 2008. "Commercializing Medicine or Benefiting the People—the First Pharmacy in China," *Science in Context* 21, 3: 311–350.

———— 2009. *The Evolution of Medicine in China: The Song Dynasty, 960–1200*. Needham Research Institution Series. London: RoutledgeCurzon.

Graham, Angus C., trans. 1981. *Chuang-tzu*. London: George Allen and Unwin.

Grant, Joanna 2003. *A Chinese Physician: Wang Ji and the "Stone Mountain Medical Case Histories."* London: Routledge Curzon.

Gujin yi'an an 古今醫案按 [Commentary on medical cases old and new]. Compiled by Yu Zhencuan 俞震篡 [Yu Dongfu 俞東扶] in 1778. Reprint, *Zhongguo yixue mingzhu* 中國醫學名著. Shenyang: Liaoning kexue jishu chubanshe, 1997.

Hsiung, Ping-chen 2007. "Facts in the Tale: Case Records and Pediatric Medicine in Late Imperial China," in Charlotte Furth, Judith T. Zeitlin, and Hsiung Ping-chen, eds., *Thinking with Cases: Specialist Knowledge in Chinese Cultural History*. Honolulu: University of Hawai'i Press, 152–168.

Hsu, Elisabeth 2010. *Pulse Diagnosis in Early Chinese Medicine: The Telling Touch*. Cambridge: Cambridge University Press.

Hu Sujia 胡苏佳 2009. "Gudai zhongyi yi'an de lishi wenhua fenxi" 古代中医医案的历史文化分析 [The historical cultural analysis of ancient Chinese medicine medical records]. Ph.D. diss., Heilongjiang Zhongyiyao daxue.

Hucker, Charles O. 1985. *A Dictionary of Official Titles in Imperial China*. Stanford, CA: Stanford University Press.

Li Jingwei 李經緯 et al. 2005. *The Great Dictionary of Chinese Medicine / Zhongyi da cidian* 中醫大辭典. 2nd ed. Beijing: Renmen weisheng chubanshe.

Liang Jun 梁峻 2004. *Zhongguo zhongyi kaoshi shi lun* 中国中医考试史论 [An essay on the history of medical examinations in China]. Beijing: Zhongyi guji chubanshe.

Liu Jingchao 劉景超 and Li Jushuang 李具雙, eds. 2006. *Xu Shuwei yixue quanshu* 許叔微醫學全書 [The complete medical works of Xu Shuwei]. Beijing: Zhongguo zhongyiyao chubanshe.

Mair, Victor H., trans. 1994. "The Biography of Hua-t'o from the History of the Three Kingdoms," in Victor H. Mair, ed., *The Columbia Anthology of Traditional Chinese Literature*. New York: Columbia University Press, 688–696.

Mattern, Susan P. 2008. *Galen and the Rhetoric of Healing*. Baltimore, MD: Johns Hopkins University Press.

Mingyi lei'an 名醫類案 [Cases of famous physicians arranged by category]. Compiled by Jiang Guan 江瓘. Preface dated 1549, first published 1591. Reprint of *Zhibuzu zhai congshu* 知不足齋叢書 ed. Beijing: Renmin weisheng chubanshe, 1957, 1982.

Mitchell, Craig, Feng Ye, and Nigel Wiseman 1999. *Shang Han Lun (On Cold Damage): Translation and Commentaries*. Brookline, MA: Paradigm.

Okanishi Tameto 岡西為人 1969. *Song yiqian yi jikao* 宋以前醫籍考 [Studies of medical books through the Song period]. 4 vols. Taibei: Ku T'ing Book House.

Puji ben shi fang 普濟本事方 [Original formulary for popular relief]. Compiled by Xu Shuwei 許叔微, 1132. Reprinted in the series *Tang Song Jin Yuan mingyi quanshu dacheng*. Beijing: Zhongguo zhongyiyao chubanshe, 2006.

Shanghan baizheng ge 傷寒百證歌 [One hundred mnemonic verses on Cold Damage manifestations]. Compiled by Xu Shuwei 許叔微, 1132. Reprinted in the series *Tang Song Jin Yuan mingyi quanshu dacheng*. Beijing: Zhongguo zhongyiyao chubanshe, 2006.

Shanghan fa wei lun 傷寒發微論 [Subtleties of Cold Damage revealed]. Compiled by Xu Shuwei 許叔微, 1132. Reprinted in the series *Tang Song Jin Yuan mingyi quanshu dacheng*. Beijing: Zhongguo zhongyiyao chubanshe, 2006.

Shanghan jiushi lun 傷寒九十論 [Ninety discussions on Cold Damage disorders]. Compiled by Xu Shuwei 許叔微, 1132. Reprinted in the series *Tang Song Jin Yuan mingyi quanshu dacheng*. Beijing: Zhongguo zhongyiyao chubanshe, 2006.

Shanghan wei zhi lun 傷寒微旨論 [Discussions on the profound meaning of Cold Damage]. Compiled by Han Zhihe 韓祇和, 1086. Reprint, *Siku quanshu*, vol. 738. Taibei: Taiwan shang wu yin shu guan, 1983.

Shanghan zabing lun 傷寒雜病論 [Treatise on Cold Damage and miscellaneous disorders]. Attributed to Zhang Ji 張機, ca. 196–220. In *Wuchang yi guan cong shu* 武昌醫館叢書, vols. 21–24. Beijing: Zhongguo shudian chuban, 1989. (The only extant version is a Ming dynasty reproduction of the Song text.)

Shennong bencao jing 神農本草經 [Divine husbandman's materia medica]. *Siku quanshu*, vol. 775. Taibei: Taiwan shang wu yin shu guan, 1983. (Late first or second century CE.)

Shi Qi 施杞 and Xiao Mincai 蕭敏材, eds. 1994. *Zhongyi bing'an xue* 中醫病案學 [The study of medical cases in Chinese medicine]. In *Bing'an xue quanshu* 病案學全書. Shanghai: Zhongguo dabaike quanshu chubanshe.

Sivin, Nathan 1967. "A Seventh-Century Chinese Medical Case History," *Bulletin of the History of Medicine* 41, 3: 267–273.

——— 1987. *Traditional Medicine in Contemporary China*. Science, Medicine, and Technology in East Asia 2. Ann Arbor: Center for Chinese Studies, University of Michigan.

——— 1995. "Text and Experience in Classical Chinese Medicine," in Don Bates, ed., *Knowledge and the Scholarly Medical Traditions*. Cambridge: Cambridge University Press, 177–204.

Skonicki, Douglas 2007. "Cosmos, State, and Society: Song Dynasty Arguments concerning the Creation of Political Order." Ph.D. diss., Harvard University.

Song ben shanghan lun 宋本傷寒論 [Song edition of the *Treatise*]. Attributed to Zhang Ji 張機, 196–220, edited by Lin Yi 林億 et al. in 1065. Reprint, Hunan: Hunan kexue jishu chubanshe, 1982.

Wang Zhengguo 王振国 2006. *Zhongguo gudai yixue jiaoyu yu kaoshi zhidu yanjiu* 中国古代医学教育与考试制度研究 [A study about the medical education and examination system in ancient China]. Jinan: Qilu shushe chubanshe.

Yan Shiyun 嚴世蕓 et al. 1990–1994. *Zhongguo yiji tongkao* 中國醫籍通考 [General compendium on traditional Chinese medical books]. 5 vols. Shanghai: Shanghai zhongyi daxue.

Yearley, Lee H. 1996. "Zhuangzi's Understanding of Skillfulness, and the Ultimate Spiritual State," in Paul Kjellberg and Philip J. Ivanhoe, eds., *Essays on Skepticism, Relativism, and Ethics in the Zhuangzi*. Albany: State University of New York Press, 152–182.

Yu Bohai 于伯海 et al. 1997. *Shanghan jinkui wenbing mingzhu jicheng* 伤寒金匮温病名著集成 [Collected famous works on Cold Damage, Golden Casket, and febrile disorders]. Beijing: Huaxia chubanshe.

Zhao Lancai 赵兰才. 2012. *Xu Shuwei yi'an ji'an* 许叔微医案集按 [Collection of Xu Shuwei's *Yi'an* with commentary]. Beijing: Huaxia chubanshe.

Zhizhai shulu jieti 直齋書錄解題 [Critical remarks on the catalog of Straightforward Studio]. Compiled by Chen Zhensun 陳振孫 (1190–1249). Reprint, Taibei: Shangwu yinshu guan, 1968.

Zhongguo yiji kao 中國醫籍考 [Studies of Chinese medical books]. Compiled by Tamba no Mototane 丹波元胤, 1819. Reprint, Beijing: Renmin weisheng chubanshe, 1983.

CHAPTER 3

Illness, Texts, and "Schools" in Danxi Medicine: A New Look at Chinese Medical History from 1320 to 1800

Fabien Simonis

Whereas the schools of Confucianism parted under the Song [960–1279], medicine split into schools in the Jin [1115–1234] and Yuan [1260–1368]…. Nevertheless, there are set principles in Confucianism but no set methods in medicine, and the circumstances of illness change in myriad ways, so it is difficult to stick to a single lineage. Hence, we shall now record the many doctrines- together.

儒之門戶分於宋　醫之門戶分於金元　　然儒有定理而醫無定法　病情萬變　難守一宗　故今所敘錄　兼眾說焉

> Preface to the section on medical works of the *Annotated Catalog of the "Complete Library of the Four Treasuries" (Siku quanshu zongmu tiyao* 四庫全書總目提要, 1798)[1]

∵

"The circumstances of illness change in myriad ways …" The notion that every instance of disease is potentially unique is so common in "traditional Chinese medicine" today that we tend to forget it has a history. The editors of the *Complete Library of the Four Treasuries (Siku quanshu* 四庫全書) adduced it to explain why they would present medical texts chronologically rather than favor one of the "schools" they claimed had fractured medical learning since the Jin and Yuan dynasties. Yet in Zhu Zhenheng's 朱震亨 (1282–1358) syncretic approach to medical doctrine this same conception of illness had been regarded

---

[1]   The citation can be found in fascicle 103 of any edition of this catalog, which its chief editor, Ji Yun 紀昀 (1724–1805), completed in 1798. I am citing from *Siku quanshu zongmu tiyao* (1798) 1999, 522.

as highly innovative. Zhu's merging of conflicting views of health and disease shaped Chinese medical thinking and writing from the late fourteenth to the late sixteenth century. The ascendancy of the "Danxi synthesis"—Danxi 丹溪 being Zhu's nickname—belies what the editors of the *Complete Library* said about scholastic divides and reminds us that the notion of illness they mentioned so matter-of-factly was not always taken for granted.

Just as the intellectual world of the Warring States period (ca. 475–221 BCE) is better understood by disregarding the "schools" into which Han dynasty (221 BCE–206 CE) scholiasts retrospectively divided it, the medical world of the late Yuan and early Ming (1368–1644) dynasties makes better sense if we do not interpret it through later classifications.[2] Below, I first explain the role of schools in the historiography of Chinese medicine. After clarifying how Zhu Zhenheng's syncretic medicine depended on a flexible notion of illness that he learned from a mentor, I explain how his disciples deployed this conception when they compiled medical treatises as montages of citations. Then I narrate how the Danxi legacy was slowly transformed in a way that de-emphasized Zhu's view of illness. Finally, I elucidate the collapse of the Danxi synthesis and the resulting invention of "Jin-Yuan medicine" and its "schools" in the seventeenth and eighteenth centuries, when this notion of illness had become so widely accepted in medical circles that critiques of Danxi forgot that Zhu Zhenheng had once been its staunchest promoter. Taken together, my arguments on conceptions of illness, forms of textual composition, and intellectual groupings (illness, texts, and schools) lead to a novel view of Chinese medical history from Zhu Zhenheng's turn to a medical career around 1320 to the compilation of the *Complete Library* a little before 1800.

"Schools" and "Currents of Learning"

The word I translate as "school" in the passage from the *Annotated Catalog* cited in the epigraph is *menhu* 門戶 (lit. "doors" or "gates"), an expression derived from pre-imperial times when pupils gathered at the gate of a master's residence to hear him lecture on specialized topics like protocol, prognostication, or poliorcetics. By the eighteenth century, as a metonym for intellectual groupings, *menhu* carried a connotation of narrowness and sectarianism. *Jia* 家, another old term, referred more neutrally either to individual "experts" or

---

2   For various critiques of the notion of "schools" as it has been applied to the pre-Han intellectual world, see van Ess 1993; Petersen 1995; Ryden 1996; Smith 2003; Csikszentmihalyi and Nylan 2003.

to "schools," the latter by extension from the character's primary meaning of "household."[3]

A more modern term for such intellectual groupings is *xuepai* 學派, which is often translated as "current of learning."[4] In the 1930s, Xie Guan (1880–1950) spoke of the "Liu Hejian current of learning" 劉河間學派 (named after Liu Wansu 劉完素, ca. 1120–1200), the "Li Dongyuan current of learning" 李東垣 學派 (after Li Gao 李杲, ca. 1180/81–1251/52), and the "Cold-Injury-learning current of learning" 傷寒學學派 (after the early third-century *Treatise on Cold Injury*, or *Treatise on Cold Damage Disorders* [*Shanghan lun* 傷寒論]).[5] Xie also accepted the claim of the *Complete Library of the Four Treasuries* that medicine had been divided into schools since at least the Jin and Yuan dynasties, a trend he deplored.[6] In his prominent textbook on Chinese medical doctrine, Ren Yingqiu cited Xie's judgment approvingly and like Xie spoke of the "Hejian" 河間, "Yishui" 易水 (named after Li Gao's master, Zhang Yuansu 張原 素, ca. 1140–ca. 1220), and "Cold Injury" currents of learning.[7]

In an influential article written in the 1990s, Wu Yi-yi tried to define the Hejian *xuepai*—a concept he translated as "group"—by mapping Liu Wansu's relations with his disciples and indirect followers from about 1200 to 1550. He made interesting finds but took for granted the existence of this "Hejian" group, perhaps because he borrowed this entity from Ren Yingqiu or perhaps because he neglected to investigate the doctrinal content of this alleged medical lineage. Besides erring on doctrinal details that should be crucial to the study of the transmission of medical knowledge, Wu also ignored the implication of the fact that all nine doctors he discusses from page 56 to page 59 read both Liu Wansu's and Li Gao's works.[8] Placing these nine doctors in Liu's intellectual

---

3   The expression "Jin Yuan si da jia" 金元四大家, for example, has been translated as either the "four great schools of the Jin and Yuan" or the "four great masters of the Jin and Yuan." For a more extensive discussion of the meaning of *jia* in Han and pre-Han scholarship, see Csikszentmihalyi and Nylan 2003, 60.

4   See Scheid 2007, 11–13.

5   See sections with these titles in Xie 1935.

6   See Xie 1935, section titled "The Transformations of Medicine" 醫學變遷, where Xie Guan paraphrases the claim of the *Annotated Catalog of the "Complete Library of the Four Treasuries."*

7   See Ren 1980, 1–2 (claim that medicine had split into schools in the Jin and Yuan periods), as well as 39, 64, and 91 (for the name of each current of learning).

8   Wu (1993–1994, 40–41) claims, for example, that Liu Wansu's "most conspicuous innovation ... was building up the *qi* of the splenetic system through the use of mainly cooling medicine." This is a surprising summary of Liu's doctrines, which emphasized the pathology of Fire rather than a particular style of replenishing. Wu (1993–1994, 41) also states that "[b]y developing Liu Wansu's point of view, [Zhang Congzheng] invented a purgation method known as *xiafa* 下法, namely, 'bringing down' by vomiting and purging."

descent is arbitrary. Choosing Li in his stead, however, would also miss the larger point that, starting in the 1320s, a number of southern doctors absorbed *both* Li's and Liu's teachings.

As it turns out, the Jin, Yuan, and early Ming, the periods to which the notion of "school" or "current of learning" was first applied—first by the editors of the *Complete Library of the Four Treasuries* and then by scholars like Xie Guan, Ren Yingqiu, and Wu Yi-yi—are the periods to which this notion applies least well. Let us now see why in more detail.

Zhu Zhenheng and Books: The Emergence of a Synthesis

Zhu Zhenheng (1282–1358) was born in Wu Prefecture—Wuzhou 婺州, soon to be renamed Jinhua 金華—a few years after the Mongols killed the last emperor of the Song dynasty (960–1279).[9] After a chivalrous though imprudent youth, in 1316 Zhu became one of the many disciples of Xu Qian 許謙 (1270–1337), a fourth-generation follower of the great Zhu Xi 朱熹 (1130–1200).[10] Despite Xu's guidance, in both 1317 and 1320 Zhu Zhenheng failed the civil examinations, which had been reestablished in 1313 with a strong emphasis on Zhu Xi's teachings.[11] He then decided to devote himself to medicine, a change of career that Xu Qian allegedly encouraged.[12]

Zhang neither invented the purgation method nor borrowed it from Liu: he took it directly from Zhang Ji's third-century *Treatise on Cold Injury*, which both he and Liu admired. This is one of the many points where Wu exaggerates the linearity of doctrinal transmission between Liu and his later admirers. Note that vomiting (*tu* 吐) was a therapeutic method distinct from *xia*, and that it was designed not to "bring down" but to expel *upward* blocked fluids that were located in the upper body.

9   Song Lian's 宋廉 "Eulogistic Epitaph of Master Danxi, Sire Zhu" 故丹溪先生朱公石表辭 (cited in *Danxi yiji* 1999, 323; hereafter "Epitaph") indicates that Zhu was born on the twenty-eighth day of the eleventh month of the eighteenth year of the Zhiyuan 至元 era, that is, January 9, 1282, of the Julian calendar.

10   Furth (2006) presents a detailed picture of Zhu's life, including his youth. Xu Qian taught in Dongyang 東陽, a few kilometers east of Zhu's native Yiwu 義烏. Both counties were part of Wu Prefecture, which was then an active center for the "Learning of the Way" 道學. For more on this region's intellectual fertility at the time, see Sun 1975; Langlois 1974, 1981; Dardess 1982, 1983; Bol 2001, 2003; Xu Yongming 2005; Chen Wenyi 2009. Song Lian ("Epitaph," 324) claims that Xu Qian had hundreds of disciples; Xu's biography in the *Yuanshi* (189.4320) speaks of more than a thousand.

11   Elman (2001, 30–38) explains the Yuan civil examinations in more detail. For a list of the works that Zhu Zhenheng studied with Xu Qian, see Simonis 2010, 109.

12   Dai Liang 戴良 (1317–1383), "Biography of the Old Man of Danxi" 丹溪翁傳 (hereafter "Biography"), in *Danxi yiji* 1999, 328.

In the last section of his *Words Bequeathed by the Ancients on the Perfection of Knowledge through the Investigation of Things* (*Gezhi yulun* 格致餘論, 1347), Zhu recounts his early medical education as a series of realizations that helped him to resolve contradictions between key medical texts.[13] Zhu's narrative of intellectual progress explains both chronologically and conceptually how he developed his syncretic approach to past medical doctrines.

At first, Zhu had admired the therapeutic precepts of Zhang Congzheng 張從正 (1156–1228), a nonconformist who had practiced medicine in the imperial capital Daliang 大梁 (Kaifeng) in the waning years of the Jin dynasty. Zhang contentiously argued that all illnesses were caused by deviant *qi* and that therapies should consist in expelling it from the body.[14] Around 1321, Zhu reread the *Basic Questions* (*Suwen* 素問)—then considered the most authoritative version of the *Yellow Emperor's Inner Canon* (first century BCE)—leaving aside dubious passages and mastering what was worth mastering (缺其所可疑 通其所可通).[15] This ability to ignore or reject parts of the medical canons would become a fundamental part of the interpretive strategy that Zhu transmitted to his disciples. After reading that the *Inner Canon* and another authority—Zhang Ji 張機 (d. 220 CE), compiler of the esteemed *Treatise on Cold Injury*—cautioned against treating depleted patients with virulent remedies, Zhu started to doubt Zhang Congzheng's universal use of aggressive therapies. The inconsistencies Zhu found between Zhang's teachings and those of the

13   That last section is titled "On Zhang Zihe's Attacking Methods" 張子和攻擊注論. I follow the editors of *Danxi yiji* (1999, 32) in replacing *zhu* 注 with *fa* 法 in the title of this section on the basis of a 1900 edition of *Gezhi yulun*. My translation of the title of the book differs from all previous ones. "Supplementary discussions" (or any variant based on the usual meaning of *yu* 餘 as "extra") is not among the attested meanings of *yulun* 餘論. See *Hanyu da cidian* 2007, 7352C; and *Grand dictionnaire Ricci de la langue chinoise* 2001 (hereafter *Grand Ricci*), entry 13219, vol. 6, 1075A. My rendering is based on the second meaning of *yulun* in those two dictionaries (前人傳留下的言論 and "propos légués par les anciens") and on the way Zhu Zhenheng explained the title in his preface: "The ancients considered medicine as one matter among classical scholars' perfection of knowledge through the investigation of things; I have therefore named these texts '*Yulun* on [the] Perfection [of Knowledge] through [the] Investigation [of Things]'" 古人以醫為吾儒格物致知一事 故目其篇曰格致餘論.

14   Zhu's summary of Zhang's precepts stayed close to the content of Zhang's *Scholar Serving His Kin* (*Rumen shiqin* 儒門事親), entry 13, "The three methods of sweating, purging, and vomiting should be able to treat all illnesses" 汗下吐三法該盡治病詮 (in *Rumen shiqin* 2.9b–13b; *Zihe yiji* 1994, 62–65). We don't know which version of Zhang's work Zhu consulted, but a three-fascicle edition of *The Scholar Serving His Kin* had been printed in 1262 (Xue 1991, 317, entry 4879).

15   Zhu made this claim in his 1347 preface to *Gezhi yulun* (*Danxi yiji* 1999, 5).

Inner Canon and the *Treatise on Cold Injury* prodded him to seek a mentor to "dispel his perplexity" 於是決意於得名師 以為之依歸 發其茅塞.[16]

When he left his native place in 1324, Zhu had studied medicine chiefly from books: the *Basic Questions*, the *Treatise on Cold Injury*, Zhang Congzheng's works, and the *Recipes of the Pharmacy Service of the Great Peace Reign* (*Taiping huimin hejiju fang* 太平惠民和劑局方), a formulary that the Song government had edited and disseminated in the twelfth and thirteenth centuries and that was still widely used in Zhu's region.[17] From his native county, Zhu traveled north on small streams until he reached the Qiantang River, which he crossed to Hangzhou and into the Wu region, where Suzhou was located.[18] "Whenever I heard that someone was practicing medicine somewhere, I would visit him to inquire" 但聞某處有某治醫 便往拜而問之. Zhu traveled north on the Grand Canal, which served as a crucial axis for the southward diffusion of northern medicine starting in the 1320s and for the northward circulation of Zhu's disciples in the second half of the fourteenth century. After going inland into Anhui, Zhu came back to the Grand Canal and proceeded north to Zhenjiang, where the Grand Canal flows into the Yangzi River. He then moved westward on the Yangzi to Nanjing. "I passed through several prefectures in succession but found no one [appropriate]" 連經數郡 無一人焉.

Though Zhu managed to obtain texts by the northern masters Liu Wansu and Li Gao that helped him to "become greatly aware of Zhang Congzheng's rashness" 乃大悟子和之孟浪, he "still had not found any conclusive discussion" 然終未得的然之議論 of the relevant doctrinal issues. Upon returning to Hangzhou in the summer of 1325 with some intriguing books but no teacher, Zhu heard of Luo Zhiti 羅知悌 (1238?–1327), an old man who had just returned from a prolonged exile in North China.[19] Zhu became his disciple in the fall.

---

16   The term *mao sai* 茅塞 (which I translate as "perplexity") was an allusion to *Mencius* 7.B.

17   In his preface to *Gezhi yulun* (*Danxi yiji* 1999, 5), Zhu claimed that he sought a teacher to understand why the formulas found in the *Recipes of the Pharmacy Service of the Great Peace Reign* could not cure the illnesses of his day.

18   My account of Zhu's travels is reconstructed from Zhu's essay on Zhang Congzheng's attacking methods (*Gezhi yulun* 67b–68a; *Danxi yiji* 1999, 32–33), Dai Liang's "Biography" (328–329), and Song Lian's "Epitaph" (326).

19   Luo was from Hangzhou, which had been the capital of the Southern Song (1127–1279). Shi Changyong (1980) argues that Luo was born around 1238. Ding Guangdi (1999, 277–280), citing the Hangzhou prefectural gazetteer, claims that Luo had served as a palace attendant under Song Lizong 理宗 (r. 1225–1264) and that when Hangzhou fell to the Mongols in 1276, the child emperor Gongzong 恭宗 (r. 1275–1276) was taken to Dadu 大都 (near modern Beijing) with his palace retinue, which included Luo. The fact that Gongzong died in 1323 (Mote 1999, 309) is consistent with the account that dates Luo

Luo was the key figure in the formation of Zhu Zhenheng's synthesis of earlier masters. In addition to being a second-generation follower of Liu Wansu, Luo was "broadly versed in the doctrines of the two experts Zhang Congzheng and Li Gao" 旁通張從正李杲二家之說 and possessed many books that Zhu had never seen.[20]

One key tenet of Luo Zhiti's teachings—and one of the "conclusive discussions" that Zhu had been seeking—was that each expert excelled at treating one kind of illness.

> Changsha [Zhang Ji's] books are detailed on external contamination, [whereas] Dongyuan [Li Gao's] books explain inner harm in detail. Only after you understand them both thoroughly can you treat illness without uneasiness.[21] If you limit yourself to the learning of Chen and Pei [Chen Shiwen 陳師文 and Pei Zongwen 裴宗文, the original compilers of the *Recipes of the Pharmacy Service*] and follow it perfunctorily, you will kill people!

> 長沙之書 詳於外感 東垣之書 詳於內傷 必兩盡之 治疾方無所 憾 區區陳裴之學 泥之且殺人

Luo Zhiti found it necessary to borrow from many masters because he conceived of illness as endlessly diverse and changing. When Zhu heard this, "his old doubts were dissipated" 夙疑為之釋然.

The widely used *Recipes of the Pharmacy Service*, which had first been compiled in the early twelfth century, recommended treating predefined illnesses with ready-made recipes. Luo taught Zhu instead that every instance of illness was unique and required a unique treatment. Indeed, Zhu claims that "there were no fixed recipes" 並無一定之方 in Luo's arsenal for the year and a half in which Zhu assisted him in seeing patients.

Zhiti's return to Hangzhou to the Taiding 泰定 reign (1324–1328). Shi (1985, 46) argues that Luo was back by 1325.

20   Dai Liang, "Biography," 329. My translation of *jia* as "experts" follows one of the renderings proposed in Csikszentmihalyi and Nylan 2003, 60. *Pangtong* 旁通 means "to be broadly versed," "to understand thoroughly" (see *Grand Ricci*, entry 8549, vol. 4, 851A; and *Hanyu da cidian* 2007, 4057B). Song Lian (who would have heard the story from Zhu Zhenheng) specified that Luo had learned Liu Wansu's medical teachings from the monk Jingshan Futu 荊山浮屠—who had purportedly been Liu's disciple—in Hangzhou during the Baoyou reign (1253–1258). See Song Lian's preface to Zhu's *Gezhi yulun*, cited in Taki (1831) 2007, 53.407.

21   One of the readings of 憾 is *dan*, which means "uneasy" (不安; *Hanyu da cidian* 2007, 4389B).

The flexible articulation of a diagnosis to a prescription is so often treated as a natural feature of "traditional Chinese medicine" that its different historical roles and the circumstances of its emergence are often neglected. Though the *Inner Canon* had often alluded to the uniqueness of each illness configuration, this view of illness did not become widespread until late imperial times. It was reemphasized by a few Song era doctors like Qian Yi 錢乙 (1026/38—1107/19)[22] and Xu Shuwei 許叔微 (1079–1154), expanded upon by the northern master Zhang Yuansu 張原素 (ca. 1140–ca. 1220), and further developed by Zhang's disciples Li Gao and Wang Haogu 王好古 (thirteenth century).[23] It is no coincidence that Luo Zhiti was "broadly versed" in Li Gao's doctrines, possessed books by Wang Haogu, and disparaged the *Recipes of the Pharmacy Service* for their inflexibility just as Zhang Yuansu and his disciples had.

After Luo Zhiti died in 1325, Zhu started taking disciples of his own. Zhu's pupils and admirers in turn became the leading transmitters of Luo's flexible art of prescription in the late fourteenth and early fifteenth centuries. Wang Xing's 王行 1377 preface to a posthumous compendium of Zhu's case files reveals how unusual Zhu's approach was seen at the time.[24] Most medical writers, Wang claimed, instructed their readers "to treat such-and-such an illness with such-and-such a remedy, and that such-and-such a remedy treats such-and-such an illness" 治某病以某方 以某方治某病而已. But "illnesses change greatly and are without constancy, whereas recipes are fixed and limited" 病多變而無常 方一定而有限. How could one "respond to inconstant illnesses with limited recipes?" 以有限之方應無常之病.[25] Wang Xing attributed these rarely-heard-of 殊不類常聞 doctrines to the aptly styled Wang Lifang 王立方 (Lifang means "establish a prescription"), who had learned them from Zhu Zhenheng's disciple Dai Sigong 戴思恭 (1324–1405).[26]

---

22   Although Qian's dates are usually given as ca. 1032–1113, we know only that he died at the age of eighty-two *sui* sometime between 1107 (the date of a preface in which Qian's admirer Yan Jizhong 閻季忠 announced that Qian was "old" and therefore alive) and 1119 (the date of Yan's posthumous publication of Qian's *Straight Secrets on the Remedies for and Disorders of Children* [*Xiaoer yaozheng zhijue* 小兒藥證直訣]).

23   For more on Zhang's views on illness, see Goldschmidt 2009, 193–197; Simonis 2010, 95–97.

24   The book was called *Danxi yi'an* 丹溪醫桉 (*Danxi's Medical Case Files* or *Danxi's Notes on Medicine*). An edition based on a manuscript copy kept at the library of the Suzhou Academy of Medicine has been published in Liu Shijue and Xue 2005.

25   Liu Shijue and Xue 2005, 3.

26   Some evidence suggests that Wang Lifang (whose real name may have been Wang Bin 王賓) stole the case records from Dai. For more on this convoluted story, see Liu Shijue, Lin, and Yang 2004, 55–56, 100–101, 194–196. Yu Bian's 俞弁 *Sequel to "Words on Medicine"* (*Xu yishuo* 續醫說, 1537; *juan* 2, entry on Wang Guang'an 王光庵) claims that when Dai moved to the Suzhou area around 1360, he was carrying "ten *juan* of medical cases [or

Contemporaneous texts explain the success of practitioners in the Danxi line by their characteristic refusal to stick to set recipes. Wang Xing attributed the "extraordinary efficacy" 奇驗 of Dai Sigong's treatments to his adoption of Zhu's flexible methods. And according to one of Jiang Wusheng's 蔣武生 (1351–1424) biographers, Jiang "did not hold to the old recipes but investigated the root of illnesses and made his own recipes; therefore, his treatments were always successful" 不執古方而究病所本 自為方 故所治恆十全.[27] Far from being taken for granted as the essence of Chinese medicine, the art of designing flexible therapies was still considered distinctive in the fifteenth century.

The spread of collections of case files 醫案 in the sixteenth century would be difficult to understand without the notion that every instance of illness deserves a unique treatment and without the prestige associated with this flexible style of prescription.[28] Interestingly, the same notion of illness also underpinned a medical genre that is usually seen as the opposite of the case collection: the general medical treatise. From a discussion of illness, we turn to one of texts.

Syncretism and the Rise of Intertextual Composition

By the 1320s, when the works of northern masters started circulating more widely in the Jiangnan region, the "Hejian," "Yishui," and "Zhongjing" currents of learning lacked the forms of social inscription, such as networks of masters and disciples, that might encourage us to call them "schools." Zhu Zhenheng was not the only physician of his time who read and thought through several of these texts. Ge Yinglei 葛應雷 (1264–1323), Ni Weide 倪維德 (1303–1377), Hua Shou 滑壽 (1304–1386), Xiang Xin 項昕 (exact dates unknown), and several others also read the works of at least two northern medical masters in the first half of the fourteenth century.[29] But Zhu was the only one who designed a coherent syncretic doctrine and transmitted it to a number of disciples who eventually wrote their own books. The precepts of important northern

---

'notes'] by [Zhu] Yanxiu [Zhenheng]" 彥修醫案十卷 (cited in Liu Shijue, Lin, and Yang 2004, 194).

27   Chen Hao 陳鎬, "Jiang Gongjing biezhuan" 蔣恭靖別傳, cited in Liu Shijue, Lin, and Yang 2004, 61–62. Late in the fourteenth century, Zhu Zhenheng's disciple Dai Sigong had recommended Jiang for the post of imperial physician, from which he eventually rose to the post of administrative assistant of the Imperial Academy of Medicine.

28   For more on the spread of case collections as a Chinese medical genre, see Cullen 2001; Furth 2007a, 2007b; Zeitlin 2007.

29   See Wu Yi-yi 1993–1994, 56–59.

physicians of the Jin and early Yuan eras (Liu Wansu, Zhang Congzheng, Li Gao, Wang Haogu, etc.) were transmitted mainly textually and through Zhu's synthesis.

Syntheses need not be made from pure forms. Zhu's syncretism borrowed from thinkers whose approaches were already synthetic in their own ways. But unlike collections of medicinal recipes from Zhu's time, which were eclectic because they assembled recipes that had been designed at different times on the basis of different understandings of illness and the body, Zhu's medicine was syncretic by design. In his own writings, he consciously re-orchestrated a variegated textual heritage into (something he presented as) a comprehensive set of medical doctrines.

The precepts that Zhu Zhenheng learned from Luo Zhiti shaped the training he gave his own disciples. Zhu's way of teaching the strengths of past specialists is evoked in an account of how he instructed Dai Sigong, who later served as the highest medical official at the Ming court in Nanjing. Zhu "selected medical books of the many experts for study. [Dai] had them all in his mind's eye: as easily as he could point to black and white, he could distinguish what was right from what was wrong and what was accurate from what was off target" 取諸家醫書讀之 了然心目間 別是非得失 若指黑白.[30] This selective appropriation of past teachings reflected Zhu's precept—which he had learned from Luo Zhiti—that all masters were right about something but not about everything. Zhu's disciples put this approach to work in their own writings.

Writing New Texts by "Synthesizing" Old Ones

Xu Yanchun 徐彥純 (d. 1384) was one of many Danxi disciples who compiled medical treatises by following Zhu's strategy of reconciling the approaches of the many masters while giving rhetorical primacy to the *Inner Canon*. Although his family was registered in the Shaoxing area (Zhejiang), Xu lived near Suzhou, where as a young scholar he taught the *Spring and Autumn Annals* to local talents.[31] In addition to a pharmacological work titled *Elaborations on Materia Medica* (*Bencao fahui* 本草發揮), Xu assembled a treatise that later commentators would refer to as the *Synthesis of Medical Learning* (*Yixue zhezhong* 醫學折衷; preface dated 1384).[32]

---

30   From Cao Chang 曹昌, "Xianyi fujun muzhiming" 顯一府君墓誌銘, Dai Sigong's epitaph.

31   Liu Chun 劉純, 1396 preface to *Subtle Meanings of the Secrets Carved in Jade* (*Yuji weiyi* 玉機微義; in Liu Chun 1999, 75).

32   This title appears in the table of contents of Liu Chun's *Yuji weiyi* (1396), a work that Liu Chun compiled on the basis of Xu's book (Liu Chun 1999, 79).

According to Liu Chun 劉純 (1340–1412), another follower of Danxi doctrines, Xu Yanchun "selected from the collected writings of Liu Shouzhen [Wansu] of the Jin and Li Mingzhi [Gao] and Zhu Yanxiu [Zhenheng] of the Yuan and synthesized (*zhezhong*) their essentials on the basis of the main precepts of the [*Inner*] *Canon*" 撅金劉守真 元李明之 朱彥修朱氏論集 本乎經旨而折衷其要.[33] Classical scholars had "synthesized" conflicting commentaries on the Classics since at least the Tang dynasty (618–907), but Liu Chun's comment on Xu Yanchun was, as far as I know, the first time a physician referred to this interpretive strategy.[34]

"Synthesis" is an approximate translation of *zhezhong* (折中 or 折衷), which could also be glossed as "balanced appraisal" or "measured judgment aiming at reconciling different views." One of *zhe*'s earliest meanings was "to break" or "to snap," both used transitively. In legal language, *zhe yu* 折獄 meant "judging [i.e., deciding] a criminal case," in which *zhe* referred not only to the trenchant aspect of a judgment but also to the weighing and pondering that led to the final decision.[35] In the terminology of textual scholarship, *zhezhong* implied the unbiased assessment of various positions available in past texts and their juxtaposition in a new entity.[36] We may also gloss *zhezhong* as to resolve a point of doctrine by arbitrating between various positions, often on

---

33   From the 1396 preface to Liu Chun's *Yuji weiyi* (Liu Chun 1999, 75). Xu probably adopted a similar approach in compiling his *Elaborations on Materia Medica*, which a sixteenth-century authority criticized because it "simply selected precepts from many masters such as Zhang Jiegu [Yuansu], Li Dongyuan [Gao], Wang Haicang [Haogu], Zhu Danxi [Zhenheng], and Cheng Wuji and combined them into one book without further additions" 取張潔古 李東垣 王海藏 朱丹溪 成無己數家之說 合成一書爾 別無增益. From Li Shizhen 李石珍, *Systematic Outline of Materia Medica* (*Bencao gangmu* 本草綱目, 1596) 1A.12a, "Lidai zhujia bencao" 歷代諸家本草, entry on *Bencao fahui* 本草發揮.

34   In the late Tang, Chen Yue 陳岳 had compiled *Synthetic Treatise on the Spring and Autumn Annals* (*Chunqiu zhezhong lun* 春秋折衷論), which survives only in fragments, to arbitrate between the Zuo, Gongyang, and Guliang commentaries to the *Spring and Autumn Annals*. As book collector and bibliographer Chao Gongwu 晁公武 (1105–1180) put it, Chen's book "compares their similarities and differences and *zhezhong*s them" 比其異同而折衷之 (see Chao's *Junzhai dushuzhi* 郡齋讀書志, cited in Hu 2009, 84).

35   *Hanyu da cidian* (2007, 1591C) glosses *zhe yu* 哲獄 as "pronouncing a sentence after detailed examination of the evidence of a case" 詳察案情而判決.

36   Taken on its own, *zhong* 衷 (fourth tone) referred to the adequacy of a decision (*Grand Ricci*, entry 2746[b], vol. 2, 272B; *Wang Li gu Hanyu zidian* 2000, 1206). Mathews (1943, 32C, char. 267) renders *zhezhong* 折衷 as "to weigh opinions; to discriminate; to compromise." See also n. 34 above.

the basis of another authority.[37] This definition is close to what Zhu Zhenheng meant when he proposed to judge the validity of contradictory statements in light of the medical classics or when he claimed more broadly that "when a multitude of sayings are in disarray, they must be judged by reference to the sages" 眾言淆亂 必折諸聖.[38]

Liu Chun's Works

Liu Chun's own treatises show how Zhu Zhenheng's syncretic approach was reinterpreted and transmitted in the late fourteenth century. Born into an illustrious family from Jiangsu, Liu first learned medicine from his father, Shu-yuan 叔淵, who may have studied with Zhu.[39] A minor master named Feng Tinggan 馮庭干 gave Liu Chun the abovementioned manuscript by Xu Yan-chun that Liu eventually expanded into the *Subtle Meanings of the Secrets Carved in Jade* (*Yuji weiyi* 玉機微義, 1396).

In the early Hongwu reign (1368–1398), Liu Chun and his family moved to the Shaanxi provincial capital Xi'an, where he practiced medicine. His first work, *Elementary Learning on the Medical Canons* (*Yijing xiaoxue* 醫經小學, 1388), aimed "to allow beginning students to [study medicine] by tracing its currents back to their source, so that they not be lured astray" 蓋欲初學者得以因流尋源 而不蹈夫他岐之惑.[40] Zhu Xi had distinguished between "lesser learning" (*xiaoxue* 小學), or the inculcation of basic skills and virtues, and "greater learning" (*daxue* 大學), or moral philosophy. In the eighteenth century, *xiaoxue* would also come to refer to philology—skills such as phonology, paleography, and glossing[41]—but in Liu Chun's work it meant two things: that the book surveyed the ideas that beginners needed to master before turning to clinical practice, and that it was a work of textual, albeit not philological, scholarship.

---

37 This corresponds roughly to the first meaning of *zhezhong* 折中 in *Hanyu da cidian* (2007, 3540C): to select evidence and use it as a yardstick for deciding on some matter (取正, 用為判斷事物的準則).

38 *Elaborations on the "Recipes of the [Pharmacy] Service"* (*Jufang fahui* 局方發揮) 22a (*Danxi yiji* 1999, 44), alluding to an almost identical passage from fascicle 2 of Yang Xiong's 楊雄 (53 BCE–18 CE) *Model Sayings* (*Fayan* 法言): 眾言淆亂則折諸聖, which Michael Nylan (2013, 37) translates as "The multitude of sayings, however contradictory, may be judged aright by reference to the sages."

39 For details on Liu's life, his origins, and his father's possible apprenticeship with Zhu Zhenheng, see Simonis 2010, 155–156, esp. 155n48.

40 See Liu Chun's preface (Liu Chun 1999, 4).

41 See Elman 2001, 207.

Julia Kristeva's claim that "any text is constructed as a mosaic of quotations" is here more literally true than she intended in her critique of Western textuality.[42] The pharmacological section of *Elementary Learning* is almost entirely based on Li Gao's writings. The first passage in the section on illness mechanisms quotes Liu Wansu's interpretation of chapter 74 of the *Basic Questions*.[43] The rest of that fascicle excerpts the *Treatise on Cold Injury*, Li Gao's *Treatise on the Spleen and Stomach* (*Piwei lun* 脾胃論), Wang Haogu's *Elementary Examples of Yin Symptoms* (*Yinzheng lueli* 陰證略例), Zhang Congzheng's *Scholar Serving His Kin* (*Rumen shiqin* 儒門事親), the *Recorded Sayings of Danxi* (*Danxi yulu* 丹溪語錄), and Zhu Zhenheng's *Words Bequeathed by the Ancients on the Perfection of Knowledge through the Investigation of Things* (*Gezhi yulun* 格致餘論).

This textual montage was no mere cut-and-paste. Liu Chun selected what he considered to be the best passages from a variety of writings that often disagreed with one another, and arranged them into a digest. It was divided into six fascicles corresponding to six branches of medicine: materia medica 本草, the pulses 脈訣, the circulation channels 經絡, illness mechanisms 病機, treatment methods 治法, and the five periods and six *qi* 運氣. Liu was one of the first writers to attempt to pack the essentials of medicine into one book.[44] To justify this doctrinal blending, Liu cited what he claimed had been Danxi's understanding of diagnosis and therapy:

> The *Inner Canon* exhausts the subtlety of yin and yang and infinite transformations: all books derive from it…. I am afraid that if one gives

---

42   See Kristeva 1986, 37.

43   Liu Wansu's interpretation had appeared in his *Method for Tracing Illnesses to Their Origin with the Mysterious Mechanism of the "Basic Questions"* (*Suwen xuanji yuanbing shi* 素問 玄機原病式, ca. 1086), a short work that Zhu Zhenheng had acquired during his quest for a teacher in the 1320s and whose content Zhu integrated—without citing it explicitly— into his influential essay "On Ministerial Fire" ("Xianghuo lun" 相火論) in *Gezhi yulun*, which I discuss below.

44   As far as I was able to determine, Zhang Yuansu's *On the Origins of Medical Learning* (*Yixue qiyuan* 醫學啟源, early thirteenth century) was the first book to adopt such a format, but this arrangement became widely imitated only in the fourteenth century and later. Wang Lü's *Tracing the Medical Canons to Their Source* (*Yijing suhui ji* 醫經溯洄集, 1368), Lou Ying's *Systematic Outline of Medical Learning* (*Yixue gangmu* 醫學綱目, 1396), Li Chan's *Introduction to Medical Learning* (*Yixue rumen* 醫學入門, 1575), Zhang Sanxi's *Six Essentials of Medical Learning* (*Yixue liuyao* 醫學六要, 1608), and Huangfu Zhong's *Enlightened Physician Pointing to His Palm* (*Mingyi zhizhang* 明醫指掌, augmented 1622 ed.) all adopted a similar structure in six sections.

primacy to Zhongjing's books and concentrates mainly on Cold Injury, one will mistake inner harm for Cold Injury. If one gives primacy to Dongyuan's books and concentrates on Stomach *qi*, I fear one will mistake external contamination for inner harm, whereas putting Hejian's books first and concentrating on Heat will lead one to mistake Cold for Heat. Instead, one should first and foremost base oneself on the *Inner Canon*: this naturally makes one alert and flexible.[45]

內經盡陰陽之妙 變化無窮 諸書皆出於此 恐先仲景書者 以傷
寒為主 恐誤內傷作外感 先東垣書者 以胃氣為主 恐誤外感為
內傷 先河間書者 以熱為主 恐誤以寒為熱 不若先主於內經 則
自然活潑潑地

Although we cannot be certain that these words were Zhu's own, they clearly represent the syncretic approach that Zhu had learned from his master Luo Zhiti. In typical *zhezhong* fashion, Liu Chun aimed to find where the teachings of the masters intersected and where they differed, the final arbiter of validity being the *Inner Canon*. The teachings of the previous masters had to be amalgamated because no single expert could exhaust the *Inner Canon* and because illnesses could not be cured by rigid adherence to any method, however excellent.

This form of doctrinal and textual synthesis was not a natural tendency of Chinese thought. The reorganization of a diverse textual legacy into florilegia purporting to present a complete and coherent picture of medicine was a novel way of composing medical texts at which several of Zhu Zhenheng's disciples excelled.

Lou Ying's *Yixue gangmu* 醫學綱目 (*1396*)
Like Xu Yanchun and Liu Chun, Lou Ying 樓英 (1320–1400) showed that writing a medical treatise required delving into a complex textual tradition.[46] He lived near Xiaoshan 蕭山, a town located southeast of Hangzhou across the Qiantang River. Probably introduced to Zhu Zhenheng by his father, Lou Youxian 樓友賢, Lou Ying studied medicine under Zhu's guidance.[47] He

---

45   Cited in "Questions on What Can Be Emulated from [the] Medical [Tradition]" ("Yi zhi ke fa wei wen" 醫之可法為問; Liu Chun 1999, 6), the extended preface to *Elementary Learning on the Medical Canons* (*Yijing xiaoxue* 醫經小學).

46   Lou's dates are those given in the Lou genealogy, which is cited in Zhou 1984.

47   Lou Youxian and Zhu Zhenheng had drunk together and exchanged poems. Some of the poems that Lou wrote on these occasions are recorded in the Lou genealogy and cited in *Danxi yiji* 1999, 714.

eventually became famous enough to be summoned to Nanjing in 1377 and 1381 to treat Zhu Yuanzhang, the founding emperor of the Ming dynasty, but he refused permanent employment at court both times.

Lou Ying started to collect materials for his summa of medical doctrines and methods in the 1360s and completed a first draft in 1380. He kept editing his text as he found more books. We can assume that his access to books was facilitated by his proximity to Hangzhou (a major cultural center with a thriving book-printing industry) and to a southern extension of the Grand Canal (a vital channel for the transmission of texts) and probably by his contacts at the Ming court in Nanjing. He achieved the final version in 1396 and called it *Systematic Outline of Medical Learning* (*Yixue gangmu* 醫學綱目).

As I have argued, composite treatises professing to cover all aspects of medicine were a new genre of medical writing in which Zhu Zhenheng's disciples specialized. These books claiming to be for beginners were in fact sophisticated digests that provided multiple points of entry into the convoluted traditions they summarized.

As an anthology of citations, the point of the *Systematic Outline of Medical Learning* was not to organize all doctrines into a perfectly rational tableau but to provide readers with a flexible repertoire of methods that would allow them to face all medical contingencies. Lou presented many possible causes for each illness, as well as an array of therapies from which physicians could choose when treating patients. What justified this catholicity was not a theoretical reflection on any particular disorder but a now-familiar one on illness in general, according to which any illness could be caused by a number of imbalances that each required a different treatment.

Recipes from any master could be effective as long as they were used to treat the kind of illness that these masters were best at curing. As Lou explained in his preface:

> Zhongjing [Zhang Ji] is detailed on external contamination that affects the interior and the surface or yin and yang. Danxi [Zhu Zhenheng] distinguishes himself on inner harm of Blood or *qi* [that causes] depletion or repletion. Dongyuan [Li Gao] supports and protects central *qi*. Hejian [Liu Wansu] removes the old to create the new. Mr. Qian [Yi] distinguishes clearly between the five yin viscera. Dairen [Zhang Congzheng] is well versed in the three methods [of vomiting, purging, and sweating]. Formularies from past ages are abundant: we can simply say that each has its strengths.[48]

---

48   "Author's preface" 自序, in Lou 1996, 2.

仲景詳外感於表裡陰陽　丹溪獨內傷於血氣虛實　東垣扶護中
氣　河間推陳致新　錢氏分明五臟　戴人熟施三法　凡歷代方書甚
眾　皆各有所長耳

This was precisely the view that Luo Zhiti had taught Zhu Zhenheng in the
1320s and that Zhu had transmitted to his disciples, except that Danxi was now
mentioned among the physicians who had practiced excellent methods that
deserved to be imitated.

The Changing Legacy of "Danxi"

For more than a century after Zhu Zhenheng's death in 1358, "Danxi medicine"
was transmitted as a synthesis of approaches, not as a specific clinical strategy.[49] Those who discussed Danxi teachings in the fourteenth and fifteenth centuries consistently depicted Zhu as a collegial thinker who had integrated the
precepts of many masters into a multifaceted approach to illness. The rise to
prominence of this body of teachings deeply shaped Chinese medical thinking
and practice in the fifteenth century.

Zhu's teachings appeared in a wide array of texts: books and manuscripts by
Zhu, notes by his disciples, works attributed to Zhu that were collated soon
after his death by people who had known him, and later "Danxi" treatises that
mixed components of these works with interpretations of what Zhu might
have thought. All these books were compiled and printed from the second half
of the fourteenth century to about 1600, when the last book attributed to Zhu
was published. I shall refer to them as the "Danxi corpus" because most of
them contained Zhu's literary name Danxi in their titles.

Sometime in the 1450s a man from Shaanxi named Yang Xun 楊珣 completed a work called *Danxi's Methods of Mental Cultivation* (*Danxi xinfa* 丹溪
心法) and had it printed in Xi'an, where Liu Chun's treatises had just been reprinted in 1439 and 1440.[50] Like Zhu's *Words Bequeathed by the Ancients on the*

---

49   See Song Lian, "Epitaph"; Dai Liang, "Biography"; the opening section of Liu Chun's 1388
      Elementary Learning on the Medical Canons; Lou Ying's 1396 preface to *Systematic Outline
      of Medical Learning*; and many more fifteenth-century sources (see Simonis 2010, chap. 5).
50   The only extant copy of Yang Xun's *Danxi xinfa* (which is held in the National Library in
      Beijing though not listed in Xue 1991) was made in Guilin in 1508 by an official who served
      there. The entire text of Yang's *Danxi xinfa* can be found in Liu Shijue and Xue 2005. For
      the translation of *xinfa* as "mental cultivation," see Elman 2001, 41. For more on Yang's
      Danxi xinfa, see Liu Shijue 1995, 112; Liu Shijue, Lin, and Yang 2004, 87–88; Liu Shijue and
      Xue 2005, 316–319.

Perfection of Knowledge through the Investigation of Things and Liu Chun's *Elementary Learning on the Medical Canons*, the title of Yang Xun's book alluded to an important concept from the "Learning of the Way," even if there was little trace of "mental cultivation" in the work itself, which was simply a digest of Danxi precepts on various maladies.[51]

Danxi's Methods of Mental Cultivation was quickly successful. Sometime after 1465, Wang Jihuan 王季瓛 republished it in Sichuan 西屬 with additional recipes.[52] Both Yang's and Wang's editions were then superseded by Cheng Chong's 程充 version, which Cheng published in Huizhou 徽州, Anhui, in 1482.[53]

In his preface to what has become the received version of *Danxi's Methods of Mental Cultivation*, Cheng explained how he had collected more Danxi recipes from a book called *A Gathering for Ordering [the World]* (*Pingzhi huicui* 平治會萃), also attributed to Zhu Zhenheng, and improved the previous editions of *Danxi's Methods of Mental Cultivation* with the help of Liu Chun's *Subtle Meanings of the Secrets Carved in Jade* (1396) and many earlier works, including books by Li Gao and Liu Wansu, two northern masters whose writings Zhu had particularly admired.

Cheng clearly recognized that Zhu's medical learning was rooted in the teachings of previous writers, but because *Danxi's Methods of Mental Cultivation* rarely cited these other masters by name, it gave the impression that Zhu had promoted his own techniques and recipes. This apparent independence helped to justify a far-reaching reinterpretation of the entire Danxi legacy.

This reinterpretation was promoted most forcefully and successfully by Wang Lun 王綸 (1453–1510; *jinshi* in 1484), a man from Cixi 慈溪 County, north of modern-day Ningbo in Zhejiang. After having served several times as provincial treasurer, he became grand coordinator 巡撫 of the important province of Huguang in 1506 but died in Suzhou a few years later.[54]

The book that made Wang Lun both famous and controversial in his own time was the *Miscellaneous Writings of Enlightened Physicians* (*Mingyi zazhu* 明醫雜著; author's preface dated 1502). In the first section of this book—titled "Of the Books of Zhongjing [Zhang Ji], Dongyuan [Li Gao], Hejian [Liu

---

51   For more details on the content of this book, see Simonis 2010, 168–169.

52   This lost edition is mentioned in Cheng Chong's 1481 preface to *Danxi xinfa* (*Danxi yiji* 1999, 137).

53   A Fujian edition is also mentioned in the "general guidelines" 凡例 of Fang Guang's 方廣 *Attached Supplements to "Danxi's Methods of Mental Cultivation"* (*Danxi xinfa fuyu* 丹溪 心法附餘, 1536), cited in Taki (1831) 2007, 53.411.

54   More on Wang's life can be found in Weng 1987.

Wansu], and Danxi, Which Are Superior?" 仲景東垣河間丹溪諸書孰優—Wang likened the *Inner Canon* to the Six Confucian Classics, and the works of these four medical masters to the Four Books, which in Wang's time were considered the most fundamental works of Confucian ethics and figured centrally in the examination system that tested candidates' grasp of the Learning of the Way.[55] Calling Zhang Ji, Li Gao, Liu Wansu, and Zhu Zhenheng the "four masters" (*sizi* 四子), Wang concluded that each was superior in treating a certain kind of illness: "for externally contracted disorders, emulate Zhongjing; for inner harm, emulate Dongyuan; for Heat illnesses, use Hejian; for miscellaneous illnesses, use Danxi; tie them up with one string: this is the complete Dao of medicine" 外感法仲景 內傷法東垣 熱病用河間 雜病用丹溪一以貫之 斯醫道之大全矣.

This interpretive move was of course typical of the syncretic strategy that Zhu Zhenheng had championed, but instead of emphasizing that Zhu had borrowed most of his therapies from his predecessors, Wang singled out the value of Zhu's methods for treating "miscellaneous illnesses," that is, anything but Cold Injury and seasonal disorders. Wang portrayed Zhu, not as a synthesizer, but as one among many masters who had a particular therapeutic strength. Zhu was thus integrated into a new synthesis in the name of the syncretic principles he had himself popularized.

Wang Lun's interpretation was plausible because "Danxi medicine" kept changing in both social coherence and doctrinal content, so that by 1500 many strains of medicine coexisted in the Danxi corpus: the approach that designed a distinct therapy for each instance of illness (which Zhu Zhenheng himself had advocated in his own writings), the Danxi who used an array of set recipes to treat clearly defined illnesses (the view implied by *Danxi's Methods of Mental Cultivation*), and the Danxi who modified a few basic remedies at bedside to fit the details of each individual case (Wang Lun's preferred version). That such dissimilar doctrines and practices could all be attributed to "Danxi" reminds us of Gérard Genette's observations that an author's name is one of the "paratexts" that shape the reading of a text or group of texts and that a single author's name may hide a great diversity of views and thus allow for dramatic reinterpretations.[56] Wang Lun's construal of Danxi was widely followed, probably because modulating ready-made recipes at bedside was much easier than designing recipes from scratch on the basis of a specific pulse diagnosis.

---

55   This subsection of Wang's work was originally untitled. Its current title is based on the first sentence of the discussion. See *Miscellaneous Writings of Enlightened Physicians*, in *Xueshi yi'an* 1997, 211.

56   Genette 1997, 37–54.

Wang also popularized the notion—still accepted today among both historians and practitioners of Chinese medicine—that Zhu specialized in "making Fire descend by nourishing yin" 滋陰降火.[57] To curb the pathological stirrings of inner Fire against which Zhu had warned in his essay "On Ministerial Fire" ("Xianghuo lun" 相火論), Wang advocated not only restraining desires and emotions but also taking protracted courses of Zhu's yin-replenishing pill 補 陰丸, a remedy composed of cooling drugs.[58] I shall not delve into the debates that Wang Lun's suggestions and his associated admonition against warming drugs soon provoked.[59] Let us simply say that critiques of Wang's cooling and yin-replenishing theories stimulated the sixteenth-century emergence of "calorific replenishing" (*wenbu* 溫補), a movement that advocated replenishing depleted vitality with *warming* drugs. As they developed and promoted new views of vitality, scholars who embraced this new therapeutic emphasis rejected what they saw as Danxi's excessive fear of Fire. Eventually, even those who opposed calorific replenishing did not return to Zhu Zhenheng's conceptions.

By 1600, "Danxi" was no longer the awe-inspiring name it had been a hundred years earlier, and the Danxi corpus no longer shaped medical debates. The declining influence of this corpus can be inferred from the dearth of editions of its key works after the mid-sixteenth century.[60] Danxi precepts had become popular partly thanks to user-friendly works like *Danxi's Methods of Mental Cultivation*, but in the seventeenth century new primers compiled by

---

57   Jutta Rall (1970, 70) treats Zhu as the founder of the "the school of fostering yin" ("die Schule des 'Yin-Förderns'"). The back cover of Yang Shou-zhong's translation (1993) of *Danxi zhifa xinyao* 丹溪治法心要 (1543) calls Zhu "the founder of the *Zi Yin Pai* or School of Enriching Yin." Zhao Pushan (1997, 160) claims that Zhu's strategy consisted mainly in "nourishing yin" and "making fire descend." Charlotte Furth (1999, 150, 162) calls "nourish Yin and make Fire descend" "Zhu's signature clinical strategy."

58   This essay can be found in Zhu's *Gezhi yulun* 56b–59b (*Danxi yiji* 1999, 28–29).

59   For more details on Wang Lun's doctrines and the reactions they elicited, see Simonis 2010, 183–190, 191–193, 214–217.

60   Copies of only one Qing edition of *Danxi xinfa* 丹溪心法 (1482) have survived in Chinese libraries; no Qing editions of *Collected Essentials of Master Danxi's Medical Books* (*Danxi xiansheng yishu zuanyao* 丹溪先生醫書纂要, 1484) and *Heart and Essentials of Danxi's Treatment Methods* (*Danxi zhifa xinyao* 丹溪治法心要, 1543) are extant. Other works embodying Danxi approaches were also disregarded: Liu Chun's *Elementary Learning on the Medical Canons* (no extant Qing ed.), Wang Lun's 王綸 *Miscellaneous Writings of Enlightened Physicians* (*Mingyi zazhu* 明醫雜著, 1502; one extant Qing ed.), Yu Tuan's 虞 搏 *The Correct Transmission of Medical Learning* (*Yixue zhengchuan* 醫學正傳, 1515; no extant Qing ed.), and Wang Ji's 汪機 *Stone Mountain's Medical Case Files* (*Shishan yi'an* 石 山醫案, 1531; one extant Qing ed., dated 1909). All these data are from Xue 1991.

Gong Tingxian 龔廷賢 (ca. 1538–1635) and Li Zhongzi 李中梓 (1588–1655) started to displace Danxi works.[61] These books remained popular into the nineteenth century.[62] We may now return to a more explicit discussion of "schools."

The New "Four Masters"

Just as the works of Danxi and other twelfth- to fourteenth-century masters stopped being reprinted, Zhang Ji's third-century *Treatise on Cold Injury* became a central focus of medical studies. One trace of the shift in prominence from Danxi to Zhang Ji was the severance of Zhang from the group of physicians with whom he had been associated since the fourteenth century. Zhu's master Luo Zhiti in the 1320s, Zhu's biographers Song Lian and Dai Liang in the 1350s, Zhu's disciples Liu Chun and Lou Ying in the last decades of the fourteenth century, and Wang Lun around 1500 had all included Zhang Ji among the specialists who had perfected therapies for one kind of disorder. Wang Lun

---

61   At least seventeen Ming and Qing editions of Gong Tingxian's *Returning to Spring after the Myriad Illnesses* (*Wanbing huichun* 萬病回春, first ed. 1587) have survived in Chinese libraries, whereas no fewer than sixty-six editions of his *Preserving the Core of Prolonging Life* (*Shoushi baoyuan* 壽世保元, first ed. 1615) were made in China between 1667 and 1911. Fifty-one editions of Li Zhongzi's *Required Readings on the Pedigree of Medicine* (*Yizong bidu* 醫宗必讀, 1637) are extant, as well as twenty-six different editions of *Three Books by Li Zhongzi* (*Shicai sanshu* 士材三書), a work that Li's Suzhou disciple You Cheng 尤乘 published twelve years after Li's death. For data, see Xue 1991, entries 04926 (*Wanbing huichun*), 4939 (*Shoushi baoyuan*), 11519 (*Yizong bidu*), and 11610 (*Shicai sanshu*).

62   *Three Books by Li Zhongzi* and Gong's *Preserving the Core of Prolonging Life* (see previous note) were two of the works that Wu Tang 吳瑭 (1758–1836) blamed his contemporaries for reading instead of the *Inner Canon* and the works of Zhang Ji. See Wu Tang, *Book for Curing the Ills of Medicine* (*Yi yi bing shu* 醫醫病書, ca. 1831), sec. 13, "On Not Reading Ancient Books" 不讀古書論; in Wu Tang 1999, 148B. Chen Xiuyuan 陳修園 (1753–1823) accused aspiring doctors of using books like Gong's *Returning to Spring after the Myriad Illnesses* as "shortcuts" 捷徑 to medical practice; he also commented that although Li Zhongzi's works "may be called shallow and rough, they hold to the constants: they are something that beginners do not dispense with" 雖曰淺率 却是守常 初學者所不廢 也. See *Three-Character Classic of Medicine* (*Yixue sanzijing* 醫學三字經, 1804), sec. 1, "The Sources and Currents of Medical Learning" 醫學源流, in that section's last entry (Chen Xiuyuan 1999, 817B); and Chen's comment on the stanza "Shicai's doctrines hold to the constants" 士材說 守其常 (Chen Xiuyuan 1999, 816B).

had called Zhang Ji, Liu Wansu, Li Gao, and Zhu Zhenheng the "four masters." Li Zhongzi renamed them the "four great experts" (*si da jia* 四大家).[63]

It was probably Suzhou physician Zhang Lu 張璐 (1617–1699) who first wrote of "the four great experts of the Jin and Yuan" (*Jin Yuan si da jia* 金元四大家), in which he replaced Zhang Ji with Zhang Congzheng (1156–1228), the advocate of aggressive therapies whom Zhu Zhenheng had admired in his youth. Zhang Lu saw Zhang Ji's doctrines as considerably superior to those of the "four great experts" and observed that Zhang Ji should not be listed among doctors he had so heavily influenced.

In a 1732 preface to one of You Yi's 尤怡 (d. 1749) many works on Zhang Ji's third-century *Treatise on Cold Injury* and *Essentials of the Golden Casket* (*Jingui yaolue* 金匱要略), Xu Dachun 徐大椿 (1693–1771) ridiculed the common belief that Zhang had specialized only in the treatment of Cold Injury and that he could be put on the same (low) footing as Liu Wansu, Li Gao, and Zhu Zhenheng.[64] Xu later developed this idea in a pugnacious assessment of the "four great experts" in his *Treatise on the Sources and Currents of Medical Learning* (*Yixue yuanliu lun* 醫學源流論, 1757). In his view, the mediocre "four great masters of the Jin and Yuan" had focused on only parts of the medical tradition. "All that [Zhu] Danxi did was ponder on the views of the various masters and arbitrate between them, subtracting here and adding there, opening a convenient and simple entry point for students" 丹溪不過斟酌諸家之言而調停去取以開學者便易之門.[65]

Just as the editors of the *Complete Library of the Four Treasuries* generally supported Han Learning, which bypassed Song scholarship on the Classics, they apparently supported Xu Dachun's dismissal of Jin and Yuan physicians and his call for returning to the *Inner Canon* and Zhang Ji's *Treatise on Cold*

---

63   *Required Readings on the Pedigree of Medicine* (*Yizong bidu* 醫宗必讀), *juan* 1, "On the Four Great Experts" 四大家論 (Li Zhongzi 1999, 80).

64   See Xu's preface to *The Heart's Canon on the Essentials of the Golden Casket* (*Jingui yaolue xindian* 金匱要略心典), in You Yi 1999, 93. Like many illustrious Qing physicians, Xu and You were from the Suzhou region.

65   And further: "Zhu's [views] are flat and simple, shallow and short-sighted; he never observed the fundamental source [of medical learning]" 朱則平易淺近 未覩本原. Both citations are from *Treatise on the Sources and Currents of Medical Learning* (*Yixue yuanliu lun* 醫學源流論, 1757), *juan* 2, "On the Four Great Masters" 四大家論 (Xu Dachun 1999, 154–155). Medical popularizer Chen Xiuyuan also adopted Zhang Lu's new interpretation of the "four masters" in his *Three-Character Classic of Medicine* (1804), dismissing Li Zhongzi's inclusion of Zhang Ji among them as "mistaken" 誤. See *Yixue sanzijing* 醫學三字經, *juan* 1, "The Sources and Currents of Medical Learning" ("Yixue yuanliu" 醫學源流), first entry (Chen Xiuyuan 1999, 816B).

Injury. They included four of Xu's works in the collection and compared Xu with Mao Qiling 毛奇齡 (1623–1716) for the ferocity of his rejection of Song and post-Song interpretations of the medical classics.[66]

Xu may indeed have been a radical antiquarian, but unlike Mao he was no textual purist. He in fact opposed attempts to reconstruct the original text (原本 or 原文) of the *Treatise on Cold Injury* and blamed Fang Youzhi 方有執 (fl. 1592) and Yu Chang 俞昌 (1585–?) for reorganizing the received version in their quest for a philologically correct edition.[67] "What is the good of disputing this great diversity of opinions when the more we interpret books by the ancients, the more abstruse they become?" 何必聚訟紛紛 致古人之書 愈講而愈晦也.[68] The text of the *Treatise* "may be jumbled and in disarray, but my heart can naturally bring everything together and thoroughly comprehend [it]" 任其顛倒錯亂 而我心自能融會貫通.[69] Xu's explanations show that a return to antiquity (*fugu* 復古) was conceivable without philological backing.

Xu Dachun presented Jin and Yuan masters as advocates of discrete and one-sided views of pathology and therapy, and Zhu Zhenheng's scholarship as derivative. Zhu's admirers had seen this syncretic derivativeness as an original solution to the problem of the infinite variety of illness, but now that Xu and most of his contemporaries, including the editors of the *Complete Library*, readily accepted the view of illness that had underpinned Zhu's medicine—Xu credited this view to Zhang Ji—they could no longer see what had made Zhu's approach distinctive in his time, notably his claim that all disorders could be cured if one borrowed from different masters the partial yet effective methods for which they were renowned. A doctrinally justified grouping of several masters who each excelled at treating one type of illness thus gave way to a chronological assemblage of biased physicians. The first grouping was the Danxi

---

66 See entry on Xu's *Treatise on the Sources and Currents of Medical Learning* in *Siku quanshu zongmu tiyao* (1798) 1999, 537.

67 Fang Youzhi's *Systematic Distinctions on the "Treatise on Cold Injury"* (*Shanghan lun tiaobian* 傷寒論條辨) was printed in 1591 after more than twenty years of effort by its author. Yu Chang completed his *Essays Exalting the "Treatise [on Cold Injury]"* (*Shang lun pian* 尚論篇) in 1648. Both Fang and Yu disparaged Wang Shuhe 王叔和 (ca. 210–285) for muddling the internal organization of the *Treatise on Cold Injury*. All editions of Zhang Ji's works since the third century have been based on Wang's reconstruction.

68 *Yixue yuanliu lun, juan* 2, "On the *Treatise on Cold Injury*" 《傷寒論》論 (Xu Dachun 1999, 150A). Cf. Unschuld 1998, 31.

69 *Yixue yuanliu lun, juan* 2, "On the *Book for Keeping People Alive*" 《活人書》論 (Xu Dachun 1999, 151B). Cf. Unschuld 1998, 328.

synthesis; the second one, "the four great experts (or schools) of the Jin and Yuan."[70]

Zhezhong and the Danxi Legacy

Paul Unschuld's widely consulted survey of Chinese medical ideas contains a brief account of "an eclectic tradition known as the School of Compromise" (*zhezhong pai* 折衷派), whose "followers did not propose any of their own theories, selecting instead those insights and instructions from the extensive medical literature that they found useful." By claiming that the adherents of this purported school shared "the concern of numerous Confucians that medical knowledge could become so highly specialized that only experts would be able to master the field," Unschuld implies that these eclectics sought to assemble a smattering of practical knowledge with little effort to integrate the results.[71]

As I have shown, *zhezhong* (which I have rendered as "synthesis" instead of "compromise") was not a lesser school of casual gleaners but the dominant interpretive strategy and mode of textual composition of Zhu Zhenheng's disciples, whose syncretic proclivities made them the most sophisticated medical writers of their age. Their reasoned collages of excerpts proposed coherent amalgamations of several therapeutic tactics. The *zhezhong* style of reasoning tried, not to produce individual claims that would be true under all circumstances, but to weave nets of statements that, taken together, would allow physicians to face any eventuality. Hinging on the notion that illness was highly diverse and constantly changing, *zhezhong* contributes to explaining why Chinese medical thinking often appears so integrative, a problem that Unschuld himself has urged historians and philosophers of science to consider seriously.

Eighteenth-century scholarship relayed by scholars from the Republican period (1911–1949) is still shaping—and, I have argued, distorting—our view of Chinese medical history. The editors of the *Complete Library of the Four Treasuries* and the countless Chinese, Japanese, and Western historians who have

---

70   My account of the origin of the "four great experts of the Jin and Yuan" differs significantly from those found in the secondary literature. See, e.g., Rall 1970; Chao 2009, 44–48. Many surveys of Chinese medical history note that Qing doctors studied the *Treatise on Cold Injury* intensively (see, e.g., Unschuld 1985, 209–210; Zhao 1997, 192–199; Li and Lin 2000, 589–596), but they are silent about how this concentration on Zhang Ji facilitated the invention of "Jin-Yuan medicine."

71   Unschuld 1985, 203.

accepted their claim about "schools" and the "four masters of the Jin and Yuan" have obscured not only the Danxi synthesis but also the textual practices and interpretive strategies of fourteenth- to sixteenth-century physicians. Only if we grasp Zhu's conscious syncretism can we explain why the most influential medical treatises from the fourteenth to the sixteenth century were anthologies of excerpts from previous texts. Their collators were guided by syncretic doctrines that they took care to present in their prefaces so that readers would appreciate their importance. These medical florilegia—the intertextual crucibles in which the late imperial understanding of most illnesses was refined— would make little sense in a medical world divided into discrete currents of learning named after individual masters.

Ironically, eighteenth-century scholars who criticized Zhu Zhenheng did exactly the same thing as Zhu in one crucial respect. "The circumstances of illness change in myriad ways, so it is difficult to stick to a single lineage," said the editors of the *Complete Library of the Four Treasuries*, an observation that Zhu would have commended. Xie Guan proposed a similar idea in his 1935 history of Chinese medicine, in which he "collected the strengths of the many doctrines and got rid of their biases and errors" 集眾說之長, 而去其偏蔽.[72] Ren Yingqiu also called upon students of Chinese medicine to master the best of each "current of learning" he presented in his introduction to Chinese medical doctrine.[73] Traditional Chinese medicine academies enact the same concept today when they emphasize the diversity of tradition and the need to adopt the best insights from each scholarly lineage. This syncretic propensity, which is now so deeply ingrained in Chinese medical thinking, finds its doctrinal roots in Zhu Zhenheng's call to borrow the best therapies from several past masters in the name of the diversity and ever-changing nature of illness.

References

Bol, Peter K. 2001. "The Rise of Local History: History, Geography, and Culture in Southern Song and Yuan Wuzhou," *Harvard Journal of Asiatic Studies* 61, 1: 37–61.

——— 2003. "Neo-Confucianism and Local Society, Twelfth to Sixteenth Centuries: A Case Study," in Paul Smith and Richard von Glahn, eds., *The Song-Yuan-Ming Transition in Chinese History*. Cambridge, MA: Harvard University Press, 241–283.

---

72   This is what Xie's disciple Qin Bowei 秦伯未 (1901–1970) praised his master for doing in the preface to Xie 1935.

73   Ren 1980, 10–14.

Chao, Yüan-ling 2009. *Medicine and Society in Late Imperial China: A Study of Physicians in Suzhou, 1600–1850*. New York: Peter Lang.

Chen Wenyi 陳雯怡 2009. "'Wu Wu wenxian zhi yi': Yuandai yige xiangli chuantong de jiangou ji qi yiyi" 「吾婺文獻之懿」—元代一個鄉里傳統的建構及其意義 ["The worthiness of our Wuzhou writings": The structure and meaning of a Yuan dynasty local tradition], *Xin shixue* 新史學 20, 2: 43–114.

Chen Xiuyuan 陳修園 1999. *Chen Xiuyuan yixue quanshu* 陳修園醫學全書 [Complete medical books of Chen Xiuyuan], edited by Lin Huiguang 林慧光. Ming-Qing mingyi quanshu dacheng. Beijing: Zhongguo Zhongyiyao chubanshe.

Csikszentmihalyi, Mark, and Michael Nylan 2003. "Constructing Lineages and Inventing Traditions through Exemplary Figures in Early China," *T'oung Pao* 89: 59–99.

Cullen, Christopher 2001. "*Yi'an* 醫案 (Case Statements): The Origin of a Genre of Chinese Medical Literature," in Elisabeth Hsü, ed., *Innovation in Chinese Medicine*. Cambridge: Cambridge University Press, 292–323.

Danxi yiji 丹溪醫集 [Collected medical writings of Danxi] 1999. 2nd ed., collated by Zhejiang sheng Zhongyiyao yanjiuyuan wenxian yanjiushi 浙江省中醫藥研究院文獻研究室. Beijing: Renmin weisheng chubanshe.

Dardess, John W. 1982. "Confucianism, Local Reform, and Centralization in Late Yuan Chekiang, 1342–1359," in William Theodore de Bary, ed., *Yuan Thought: Chinese Thought and Religion under the Mongols*. New York: Columbia University Press, 327–374.

——— 1983. *Confucianism and Autocracy: Professional Elites in the Founding of the Ming Dynasty*. Berkeley: University of California Press.

Ding Guangdi 丁光迪, ed. 1999. *Jin-Yuan yixue pingxi* 金元醫學評析 [Critical analysis of Jin-Yuan medicine]. Beijing: Renmin weisheng chubanshe.

Elman, Benjamin A. 2001. *From Philosophy to Philology: Intellectual and Social Aspects of Change in Late Imperial China*, 2nd, rev. ed. UCLA Asian Pacific Monograph Series. Los Angeles: University of California Press.

Furth, Charlotte 1999. *A Flourishing Yin: Gender in China's Medical History, 960–1665*. Stanford, CA: Stanford University Press.

——— 2006. "The Physician as Philosopher of the Way: Zhu Zhenheng (1283–1358)," *Harvard Journal of Asiatic Studies* 66, 2: 423–459.

——— 2007a. "Introduction: Thinking with Cases," in Furth, Zeitlin, and Hsiung 2007, 1–27.

——— 2007b. "Producing Medical Knowledge through Cases: History, Evidence, and Action," in Furth, Zeitlin, and Hsiung 2007, 125–151.

Furth, Charlotte, Judith Zeitlin, and Hsiung Ping-chen, eds. 2007. *Thinking with Cases: Specialist Knowledge in Chinese Cultural History*. Honolulu: University of Hawai'i Press.

Genette, Gérard 1997. *Paratexts: Thresholds of Interpretation*, translated by Jane E. Lewin. Cambridge: Cambridge University Press. Originally published as *Seuils* (Paris: Seuil, 1987).

Goldschmidt, Asaf 2009. *The Evolution of Chinese Medicine: Song Dynasty, 960–1200*. New York: Routledge.

Grand dictionnaire Ricci de la langue chinoise 2001. Paris and Taibei: Instituts Ricci and Desclée de Brouwer.

Hanyu da cidian 漢語大詞典 [Great dictionary of Chinese] 2007. Suoyin ben 縮印本 [Small-print ed.]. Compiled by *Hanyu da cidian* bianji weiyuanhui 《漢語大詞典》編輯委員會 (edited by Luo Zhufeng 羅竹風) and *Hanyu da cidian* bianzuan chu 《漢語大詞典》編纂處, 3 vols. Shanghai: Shanghai cishu chubanshe.

Hu Chusheng 胡楚生 2009. "Chen Yue *Chunqiu zhezhong lun* xiping" 陳岳《春秋折衷論》析評 [Critical analysis of Chen Yue's *Synthetic Treatise on the Spring and Autumn Annals*], *Jingxue yanjiu jikan* 經學研究集刊 6: 83–92.

Kristeva, Julia 1986. "Word, Dialogue, and the Novel," in T. Moi, ed., *The Kristeva Reader*. New York: Columbia University Press, 35–61. Originally published as "Le mot, le dialogue et le roman," in *Recherches pour une sémanalyse* (Paris: Seuil, 1969).

Langlois, John D., Jr. 1974. "Chin-hua Confucianism under the Mongols (1279–1368)." Ph.D. diss., Princeton University.

——— 1981. "Political Thought in Chin-hua under Mongol Rule," in John D. Langlois Jr., ed., *China under Mongol Rule*. Princeton, NJ: Princeton University Press, 137–185.

Li Jingwei 李經緯 and Lin Zhaogeng 林昭庚, eds. 2000. *Zhongguo yixue tongshi* 中國醫學通史 [General history of Chinese medicine], *Gudai juan* 古代卷 [Ancient (China) volume]. Beijing: Renmin weisheng chubanshe.

Li Zhongzi 李中梓 1999. *Li Zhongzi yixue quanshu* 李中梓醫學全書 [Complete medical books of Li Zhongzi], edited by Bao Laifa 包來發. Ming-Qing mingyi quanshu dacheng. Beijing: Zhongguo Zhongyiyao chubanshe.

Liu Chun 劉純 1999. *Liu Chun yixue quanshu* 劉純醫學全書 [Complete medical books of Liu Chun], edited by Jiang Dianhua 姜典華. Ming-Qing mingyi quanshu dacheng 明清明醫全書大成. Beijing: Zhongguo Zhongyiyao chubanshe.

Liu Shijue 劉時覺 1995. "*Danxi xinfa* ji Zhushi xiangguan zhuzuo kao" 《丹溪心法》及朱氏相关著作考 [Inquiry on *Danxi's Methods of Mental Cultivation* and Zhu Zhenheng's related works], *Zhonghua yishi zazhi* 中華醫史雜誌 25, 2: 111–113.

Liu Shijue, Lin Qianliang 林乾良, and Yang Guanhu 楊觀虎, eds. 2004. *Danxi xue yanjiu* 丹溪學研究 [Research on Danxi learning]. Beijing: Zhongyi guji chubanshe.

Liu Shijue and Xue Yiyan 薛轶燕, eds. 2005. *Danxi yishu* 丹溪逸书 [Lost books by Danxi]. Shanghai: Shanghai Zhongyiyao daxue chubanshe.

Lou Ying 樓英 (1396) 1996. *Yixue gangmu* 醫學綱目 [Systematic outline of medical learning]. Beijing: Zhongguo Zhongyiyao chubanshe.

Mathews, R. H. 1943. *Mathews' Chinese-English Dictionary*, rev. American ed. Cambridge, MA: Harvard-Yenching Institute.

Mote, Frederick W. 1999. *Imperial China: 900–1800*. Cambridge, MA: Harvard University Press.

Nylan, Michael, trans. 2013. *Exemplary Figures: Fayan* 法言. Seattle: University of Washington Press.

Petersen, Jens Østergård 1995. "Which Books Did the First Emperor of Ch'in Burn? On the Meaning of Bai Chia in Early Chinese Sources," *Monumenta Serica* 43: 1–52.

Rall, Jutta 1970. *Die vier grossen Medizinschulen der Mongolenzeit: Stand und Entwicklung der chinesischen Medizin in der Chin- und Yuan-Zeit*. Wiesbaden: Franz Steiner Verlag.

Ren Yingqiu 任應秋 1980. *Zhongyi gejia xueshuo* 中醫各家學說 [The doctrines of the various schools of Chinese medicine]. Shanghai: Shanghai kexue jishu chubanshe.

Ryden, Edmund 1996. "Was Confucius a Confucian? Confusion over the Use of the Term 'School' in Chinese Philosophy," *Early China News* 9: 5–9, 28–29.

Scheid, Volker 2007. *Currents of Tradition in Chinese Medicine, 1626–2006*. Seattle: Eastland Press.

Shi Changyong 史常永 1980. "Luo Zhiti shengping zhushu ji *Luo Taiwu xiansheng koushou sanfa* kao" 羅知悌生平著述及《羅太無先生口授三法》考 [On the life and works of Luo Zhiti, with an investigation of *The Three Methods Taught Orally by Master Luo Taiwu*], *Zhonghua yishi zazhi* 中華醫史雜誌 10, 1.

——— 1985. "Luo Zhiti zhuan gao" 羅知悌傳稿 [Draft biography of Luo Zhiti], *Shanghai Zhongyiyao zazhi* 上海中医药杂志 1985, 6: 46–47.

Siku quanshu zongmu tiyao 四庫全書總目提要 [Annotated catalog of the *Complete Library of the Four Treasuries*] (1798) 1999. Originally compiled by Yongrong 永瑢 and Ji Yun 紀昀, modern ed. collated by the *Siku quanshu zongmu tiyao* Editing Committee 四庫全書總目提要編委會. Haikou: Hainan chubanshe.

Simonis, Fabien 2010. "Mad Acts, Mad Speech, and Mad People in Late Imperial Chinese Law and Medicine." Ph.D. diss., Princeton University.

Smith, Kidder 2003. "Sima Tan and the Invention of 'Daoism,' 'Legalism,' et cetera," *Journal of Asian Studies* 62, 1: 129–156.

Sun Kekuan 孫克寬 1975. *Yuandai Jinhua xueshu* 元代金華學術 [Scholarship in Yuan dynasty Jinhua]. Taizhong: Donghai daxue chubanshe.

Taki Mototane 多紀元胤 (also known as Tamba no Mototane 丹波元胤) (1831) 2007. *Iseki kō* 醫籍考 [Research on (Chinese) medical books], 80 *juan*. Beijing: Xueyuan chubanshe. Arranged by Guo Xiumei 郭秀梅 and Okada Kenkichi 岡田研吉, based on Fujikawa Yū's 富士川遊 photoreproduction of the handwritten original (Tokyo: Kokuhon shuppansha, 1935). Often cited as *Zhongguo yiji kao* 中國醫籍考, the title adopted by Renmin weisheng chubanshe for their 1983 ed.

Unschuld, Paul U. 1985. *Medicine in China: A History of Ideas*. Comparative Studies of Health Systems and Medical Care. Berkeley: University of California Press.

———— 1998. *Forgotten Traditions of Ancient Chinese Medicine: The "I-Hsüeh Yüan Liu Lun" of 1757 by Hsü Ta-ch'un*. Brookline, MA: Paradigm Publications.

van Ess, Hans 1993. "The Meaning of Huang-Lao in *Shiji* and *Hanshu*," *Études chinoises* 12, 2: 161–177.

Wang Li gu Hanyu zidian 王力古漢語字典 [Wang Li's dictionary of ancient Chinese] 2000. Compiled under the direction of Wang Li 王力. Beijing: Zhonghua shuju.

Weng Fuqing 翁福清 1987. "Wang Lun muzhiming jieshao" 王綸墓誌銘介紹 [A presentation of Wang Lun's epitaph], *Zhejiang Zhongyi zazhi* 浙江中醫雜誌 22, 9.

Wu Tang 吳瑭 1999. *Wu Jutong yixue quanshu* 吳鞠通醫學全書 [Complete medical books of Wu Jutong], edited by Li Liukun 李劉坤. Beijing: Zhongguo Zhongyiyao chubanshe.

Wu Yi-yi 1993–1994. "A Medical Line of Many Masters: A Prosopographical Study of Liu Wansu and His Disciples from the Jin to the Early Ming," *Chinese Science* 11: 36–65.

Xie Guan 謝觀 1935. *Zhongguo yixue yuanliu lun* 中國醫學源流論 [On the sources and currents of Chinese medicine]. Shanghai: Shanghai Zhongyi shuju.

Xu Dachun 徐大椿 1999. *Xu Lingtai yixue quanshu* 徐靈胎醫學全書 [Complete medical books of Xu Lingtai], edited by Liu Yang 劉洋. Ming-Qing mingyi quanshu dacheng. Beijing: Zhongguo Zhongyiyao chubanshe.

Xu Yongming 徐永明 2005. *Yuandai zhi Mingchu Wuzhou zuojiaqun yanjiu* 元代至明初婺州作家群研究 [Research on Wuzhou writers in the late Yuan and early Ming]. Beijing: Zhongguo shehui kexue chubanshe.

Xue Qinglu 薛清錄, ed. 1991. *Quanguo Zhongyi tushu lianhe mulu* 全國中醫圖書聯合目錄 [National union catalog of Chinese medical books], compiled by Zhongguo Zhongyi yanjiuyuan tushuguan 中國中醫研究院圖書館. Beijing: Zhongyi guji chubanshe.

Xueshi yi'an 薛氏醫案 [Mr. Xue's medical case files (or, Mr. Xue's notes on medicine)] 1997. Beijing: Zhongguo Zhongyiyao chubanshe.

Yang Shou-zhong, trans. 1993. *The Heart and Essence of Dan-Xi's Methods of Treatment: A Translation of Zhu Dan-Xi's Zhi Fa Xin Yao*. Boulder, CO: Blue Poppy Press.

You Yi 尤怡 1999. *You Zaijing yixue quanshu* 尤在涇醫學全書 [Complete medical books of You Zaijing], edited by Sun Zhongtang 孫中堂. Ming-Qing mingyi quanshu dacheng. Beijing: Zhongguo Zhongyiyao chubanshe.

Yuanshi 元史 [History of Yuan] 1370. Compiled by Song Lian 宋濂. Beijing: Zhonghua shuju.

Zeitlin, Judith T. 2007. "The Literary Fashioning of Medical Authority: A Study of Sun Yikui's Case Histories," in Furth, Zeitlin, and Hsiung 2007, 169–202.

Zhao Pushan 趙璞珊 1997. *Zhongguo gudai yixue* 中國古代醫學 [Medicine in ancient China]. Beijing: Zhonghua shuju.

Zhou Mingdao 周明道 1984. "Mingdai yixuejia Lou Ying nianbiao" 明代醫學家樓英
    年表 [Chronology of the Ming dynasty physician Lou Ying], *Zhonghua yishi zazhi*
    中華醫史雜誌 14, 3: 154.

Zihe yiji 子和醫集 [Collected medical writings of Zihe (i.e., Zhang Congzheng)] 1994.
    Edited by Deng Tietao 鄧鐵濤. Beijing: Renmin weisheng chubanshe.

CHAPTER 4

Ancient Texts and New Medical Ideas in Eighteenth-Century Japan

Daniel Trambaiolo

Introduction

The early eighteenth century in Japan witnessed a broad transformation of intellectual attitudes and practices that altered basic assumptions about the nature of evidence and interpretation in fields as diverse as classical studies,
astronomy, medicine, and natural history.[1] As one of the most socially presti-
gious and intellectually sophisticated models of evidential argument, critical
textual philology played a central role in this transformation: beginning in the
late seventeenth century, Confucian philologists such as Itō Jinsai 伊藤仁齋
(1627–1705) and Ogyū Sorai 荻生徂徠 (1666–1728) had begun to reject traditions of philosophical interpretation that had shaped readings of the classics
since the Song dynasty, seeking instead to rediscover these classics' original
significance through the close study of "ancient meanings" (*kogi* 古義) and
"ancient phraseology" (*kobunji* 古文辭).[2] The "Ancient Formulas" (*koho* 古方)
doctors of the eighteenth century sought to bring about a parallel transformation in the understanding and practice of medicine, criticizing orthodox medical styles that had developed since the Song dynasty as the degenerate
medicine of a "Later Age" (*gosei* 後世) and basing their therapies instead on
the writings of the second-century Chinese doctor Zhang Zhongjing 张仲景.[3]

One paradoxical consequence of this attempt to restore the medicine of antiquity was the development of an entirely new approach to the epistemic
foundations of medicine that combined direct observation with the philological study of early texts.[4] Yoshimasu Tōdō 吉益東洞 (1702–1773) and Yamawaki
Tōyō 山脇東洋 (1705–1762), two of the most influential Ancient Formulas doc-

---

1   Kasaya 2011.

2   Yoshikawa 1983. On the contemporaneous intellectual shift "from philosophy to philol-
    ogy" in China, see Elman 2001.

3   Kure 1918, 5; Fujikawa 1941, 296–299, 342–366, 429–433; Sugimoto and Swain 1978, 280–
    284; Kosoto 1999, 153–158; Aoki 2012, 69–93.

4   Yamada 1997; Machi 1998a, 1998b; Tateno 2004; Yamada 2006; Terasawa 2012.

© KONINKLIJKE BRILL NV, LEIDEN, 2015 | DOI 10.1163/9789004285453_005

tors of the eighteenth century, drew on the ideas and rhetoric of Ogyū Sorai to argue that the study of "ancient words" should supplement the study of "ancient techniques," because "by the words one knows the age and by the techniques one knows the people," and searched extensively through the corpus of surviving ancient literature for passages that might yield insights into the medicine of Chinese antiquity.[5] Rather than seeking to substitute their own observations for the authority of texts, they undertook their empirical investigations in the confidence that these investigations would support the conclusions of their philological scholarship.

This desire to restore the medicine of antiquity through textual and practical investigations was intimately linked to the Ancient Formulas doctors' ongoing struggle to define an appropriate social and intellectual status for themselves as elite practitioners of the art of medicine. Together with the intellectual example of Confucian philology, the character of medical practice in the urban society of eighteenth-century Japan thus forms an essential basis for understanding the Ancient Formulas doctors' most characteristic contributions to the later development of Tokugawa medicine, including Yamawaki Tōyō's investigations into human anatomy and Yoshimasu Tōdō's arguments about the nature of drug therapies.

Textual Learning and Medical Knowledge in Tokugawa Society

By the beginning of the eighteenth century, the spread of literacy, the growth of the publishing industry, and the proliferation of schools and academies had helped transform the ability to understand classical Chinese texts from a rare skill possessed by a few specialists to an educational foundation desirable for a wide range of social groups. At the same time, these changes helped a growing number of individuals gain access to medical learning through the medium of written texts, and the social characteristics of classical scholarship and medical learning thus evolved in parallel.[6] Prominent seventeenth-century scholarly doctors such as Hori Kyōan 堀杏庵 (1585–1642), Emura Sensai 江村專齋 (1565–1664), and Mori Unchiku 森雲竹 (1631–1712) established a pattern of combining the practice of medicine with the study of the Confucian classics, and Ujita Un'an 宇治田雲庵 (1618–1686), a doctor in the service of Wakayama domain, argued that medical cultivation of the body and Confucian cultiva-

---

5   Yamawaki Tōyō 1751, 9a. See also Yamawaki Tōyō 1751, 7a; 1759, 1:26b–27a, 2:17b–18a.
6   Rai 1993; Yokota 1998; Kornicki 1998, 258–276; Rubinger 2007, 9–43; Trambaiolo 2014b.

tion of the self were complementary aspects of the same Way.[7] Broad study of the Chinese classics offered a path to better understanding of the ancient texts from which medical learning derived, while the practice of medicine represented a way for aspiring scholars to earn a living while they pursued financially unprofitable studies of Chinese texts. For many doctors who considered themselves members of the medical elite, medical and scholarly activities thus came to form a single continuous field of cultural practice.[8]

Reacting against the increasingly widespread combination of medicine and Confucian scholarship, Itō Jinsai criticized the very concept of "Confucian doctors" (*jui* 儒醫), declaring that medicine was an affair for "petty people" (*shōjin* 小人) and that so-called "Confucian doctors" were merely doctors who sought to attract patients and profits through unjustifiable claims of erudition.[9] Early eighteenth-century scholars and doctors such as Ogyū Sorai, Dazai Shundai 太宰春台 (1680–1747), and Naitō Kitetsu 内藤希哲 (1701–1735) adopted views similar to those of Jinsai concerning the fundamentally distinct characteristics of medicine and Confucian learning.

Nevertheless, polemics against "Confucian doctors" were fully compatible with the assumption that doctors needed to cultivate many of the same linguistic and philological skills as Confucians. Dazai Shundai lamented the fact that because the most philologically gifted students tended to become Confucian scholars rather than doctors, many of those who did become doctors never mastered the study of ancient phraseology to the extent necessary for serious study of the medical classics.[10] Even some of Jinsai's own disciples insisted on the desirability of combining Confucian study and medical practice: Namikawa Tenmin 並河天民 (1679–1718), for example, actively encouraged Japanese Confucian scholars to practice medicine in order to have a means of financial support.[11] Whether for intellectual or for purely pragmatic reasons, many individuals chose to cultivate simultaneous double identities as doctors and Confucian scholars.

---

7   Ujita 1681, quoted in Lan 2007, 78.

8   For a biographical and intellectual survey of scholar-doctors who combined Confucian learning and medicine during the Tokugawa period, see Anzai 1943.

9   Hattori 1978, 28–29. For a survey of Jinsai's relationships with doctors, see Hattori 1978, 44–54. Yoshikawa Kōjirō (1983, 73) has suggested that Jinsai's views on this issue may have had their basis in his biography, since Jinsai had refused to follow his relatives' advice to take up the practice of medicine as his own occupation. Jinsai's warnings that Confucian scholars should not become involved in medicine continued to be taken seriously as late as the mid-nineteenth century: for an example, see Macé 1997, 408.

10   Hattori 1978, 63.

11   Hattori 1978, 27–34.

From the early eighteenth century onward, advocates of Ancient Formulas medicine took an active interest in these debates concerning the social status of medical learning and medical practitioners. Gotō Konzan 後藤艮山 (1659–1733) noted that Zhang Zhongjing himself had been a government official in the service of the Han dynasty and thus was not a "doctor" in the sense of having had medicine as his occupation. Konzan suggested that medicine should not be thought of as an occupation (*gyō* 業) but simply as the art of treating the sick, arguing that doctors who viewed medicine as an occupation tended to become excessively focused on cultivating fame and profit.[12] Yamawaki Tōyō wrote that both in China and in Japan, medicine had been pursued as an easy path to profit by people lacking in literary or military talent and with insufficient land or money to make a living through farming or trading, and both he and Yoshimasu Tōdō consistently referred to medicine as a "humble occupation" (*sengyō* 賤業, *senshoku* 賤職).[13] Tōyō's disciple Nagatomi Dokushōan 永富獨嘯庵 (1732–1766) was best known as a doctor, but his nephew took pains to point out that the practice of medicine did not constitute his "essential character" (*honshoku* 本色), and when Dokushōan's disciple Kamei Nanmei 龜井南冥 (1743–1814) met with representatives of a visiting Korean embassy, he was at least as eager to praise his teacher's scholarly and literary writings as his medical ideas.[14] Kagawa Shūan 香川修庵 (1683–1755), a disciple of Itō Jinsai, disregarded Jinsai's criticisms of Confucian doctors and declared that "Confucianism and medicine have a single root" (*ju i ippon* 儒醫一本); later advocates of Ancient Formulas pointed out that this idea could provide valuable moral support to sons of hereditary medical families, who often felt ashamed to engage in an occupation whose practitioners were notorious for their lack of scholarship.[15] These remarks suggest that many advocates of Ancient Formulas medicine felt embarrassed about the low prestige of their profession, and their efforts to develop new styles of medical scholarship modeled on contemporary currents of Confucian learning may have been prompted by a desire to compensate for this sense of inferiority.

Yoshimasu Tōdō's ambivalent statements about his own status as a doctor offer particularly revealing glimpses into the nature of the social, cultural, and

---

12   Gotō (n.d.) 1971, 390–392.

13   Yamawaki Tōyō 1751, 24b. Cf. Yamawaki Tōyō 1751, 5a–b, 18a, 32a, 33b; 1759, 1:23b; (n.d.) 1979, 409; Yoshimasu (1800) 1918e, 503. For discussion, see Yamada 1997, 479–482.

14   Nagatomi (1764) 1807, preface by Fuji Takaaki 藤隆昌; Kamei 1764. For further discussion of the medical dialogues held in the context of embassies from Chosŏn Korea to Tokugawa Japan, see Trambaiolo 2014a.

15   Kagawa 1744, preface by Suga Akira 菅斐, 1a. On Kagawa's idea that Confucianism and medicine had a single root, see also Machi 1998a.

psychological tensions surrounding the status of medical practitioners. Tōdō admitted to one correspondent that he thought of medicine as no more than "a technical skill and a humble profession," and he later wrote that "even the name 'doctor' is shameful."[16] Nevertheless, Tōdō also took pride in his occupation, believing that medicine should be practiced as a primary duty (*honshoku* 本職) rather than regarded as a field of learning that scholars could acquire and practice casually.[17]

Tōdō's ambivalence about his own status as a doctor can be seen most clearly in his description of a dream he claimed to have had soon after his arrival in Kyoto, when his financial problems and the difficulty he experienced in attracting patients had forced him to earn a living by making and selling dolls. Tōdō dreamed of an argument between a clay doll and a wooden doll in which each doll proclaimed its own superiority on the basis of the material from which it was made; the two dolls continued to argue inconclusively until they were interrupted by a paper doll, who pointed out that both sides of the debate were founded on a mistaken assumption about the relationship between innate nature and social function:

> The uprightness of wood and the simple honesty of earth are their Heaven-bestowed natures (*tensei* 天性). Clay is clay and wood is wood, and they cannot be substituted for one another. It is the same with people. Human nature (*jinsei* 人性) is many-sided, and each person possesses some merits while lacking others. Since this is the case, people should satisfy their Heaven-bestowed natures and fulfill their Heaven-bestowed duty (*tenshoku* 天職).... We are born through the command of Heaven (*tenmei* 天命), and we should strive to make use of what we have received from Heaven; to strive without ceasing is to accept our Heaven-bestowed duty.[18]

Tōdō and Tōyō saw their pursuit of scholarly learning as an integral aspect of their social function as medical practitioners, and they therefore sought to familiarize themselves with the ideas and methods of contemporary scholars

---

16   Yoshimasu (1800) 1918e, 503; (1825) 1918g, 575.

17   Yoshimasu (1814) 1918f, 55.

18   Yoshimasu (1800) 1918e, 513. Tōdō's description of this dream is found in a letter he wrote to the Confucian scholar Udono Shinei 鵜殿士寧 (1710–1774), a disciple of Hattori Nankaku whom Tōdō admired as an authority on statecraft (*keizai* 経済); although the letter is not dated, the implicit message that Tōdō's difficulties were well behind him at the time of writing suggests that it was written no earlier than ca. 1750 and perhaps much later.

of Chinese learning and to develop analogous ideas and methods in their own field.

Ogyū Sorai and Ancient Formulas Medicine

Ogyū Sorai was one of the most influential intellectual figures of eighteenth-century Japan, renowned for his literary, philological, and philosophical writings.[19] Sorai's approach to understanding the Confucian classics was premised on his conviction that the meanings of early Chinese texts should be discerned through the evidential study of ancient language and phraseology rather than by reference to intuitively comprehended moral principles. Similarly, he proposed that the Way of the Ancient Kings (*sennō no michi* 先王之道) had been about "things" (*mono/butsu* 物) rather than Principle (*ri* 理), and he argued that the Ancient Kings' achievements derived not from their superior moral natures but from the practical "techniques" (*waza/jutsu* 術) they had employed and bequeathed to later generations.[20] His moral and political philosophy thus emphasized the importance of concrete forms of social organization, insisting that it was a mistake to think of the Way as having an existence independent of its embodiment in rites, music, punishments, and governance.[21]

These ideas had a sensational impact on Japanese intellectual culture during the middle years of the eighteenth century. They were rapidly disseminated through the medium of printed books, and their reception thus extended to all readers who were willing to approach the challenges presented by Sorai's innovative ideas and his often intricate *kanbun* prose.[22] Nawa Rodō 那波魯堂 (1727–1789), a critic of Sorai and a defender of Zhu Xi's ideas, later recalled that popular enthusiasm for Sorai's ideas "was most extreme for a period of twelve or thirteen years from Genbun through to Enkyō and Kan'en [1736–1750], when people studied and rejoiced in his doctrines as if they had truly gone mad."[23]

Many doctors joined in with this enthusiasm. Yamawaki Tōyō described his initial contact with Sorai's writings as a thrilling encounter, commenting: "I was almost forty years old when I first obtained Sorai's books, but in reading

---

19   The literature on Ogyū Sorai is too extensive to summarize here; my account here draws
      selectively on Maruyama 1974; Yoshikawa 1983; Najita 1998; Tucker 2006; Flueckiger 2011;
      Bitō 2013. For discussion of Sorai's writings on medicine, see Hattori 1978, 54–62; Lan 2007.
20   Ogyū (1717) 1973a, 26, 28–30, 205, 206.
21   Ogyū (1717) 1973a, 13, 201; (1727) 1973c, 304–306.
22   Nakamura 1996, 43.
23   Nakamura 1996, 32.

them I became exhilarated to the point of forgetting myself. It was like gazing on the great ocean. The more I read, the more I believed, and though the day turned to night, I experienced no fatigue."[24] When Tōyō traveled to Edo in 1746 to present his new edition of Wang Tao's *Medical Secrets from the Royal Library* (*Waitai miyao fang* 外臺秘要方) to the *bakufu*, he regarded the opportunity to meet Sorai's disciples Dazai Shundai and Hattori Nankaku 服部南郭 (1683–1759) as a highlight of the journey.[25]

Sorai's ideas thus came to play a crucial role in shaping the character of Ancient Formulas medicine for Japanese doctors during the middle decades of the eighteenth century, when Yamawaki Tōyō and Yoshimasu Tōdō drew parallels between their own aim of restoring the medicine of antiquity and Sorai's aim of restoring the original meanings of the Confucian classics. Sorai's writings were not the initial stimulus for the emergence of Ancient Formulas medicine itself—Nagoya Gen'i 名古屋玄医 (1628–1696) and Gotō Konzan, inspired in part by the writings of Chinese doctors such as Fang Youzhi 方有執 (1523–1593), Yu Jiayan 喻嘉言 (1585–1684), and Cheng Yingmao 程應旄, had been advocating revival of Zhang Zhongjing's formulas several decades before Sorai's ideas became widely known—but Tōdō's and Tōyō's recognition of the analogies between Sorai's aims and their own provided them with a powerful set of concepts and methods for developing their distinctive style of medical thought and practice.

One of Sorai's central objections to orthodox Neo-Confucian philosophy was his claim that it had departed from the correct uses of language by concerning itself with abstract "Principle" rather than concrete "things," producing an empty discourse that distorted the proper relationships between language and reality. Tōdō and Tōyō adapted this rhetoric to develop a parallel argument against the conceptual basis of "Later Age" medicine. In criticizing the philosophical centrality of Principle in the writings of Song Neo-Confucians, Sorai had written that "Principle has no form (*katachi/kei* 形) and thus has no standards (*jun* 準).... Different people see things differently.... It is like when two peasants are disputing a property boundary—if there is no official to hear the dispute, what can serve as a standard?"[26] Yoshimasu Tōdō borrowed directly from these arguments to support his critique of the excessively abstract character of orthodox medical discourse: "Principle has no fixed standards (*jun* 準), while diseases have fixed symptoms (*shō* 證). How can we use Principle with-

---

24   Yamawaki Tōyō 1759, 2:20b.
25   Yamawaki Tōyō 1751, 22a–b; 1759, 2:17a–21a.
26   Ogyū (1717) 1973a, 28, 206; cf. Ogyū (1717) 1973b, 150, 244.

out fixed standards to confront diseases with fixed symptoms?"[27] Yamawaki Tōyō's allusions to Sorai were no less clear: "Principle can be turned upside down, but how can things (*mono* 物) be mistaken? If we treat Principle as primary and things as secondary, then even the most intelligent people cannot avoid error."[28]

Sorai's own views of the appropriate relationship between doctors and society can be found in his late unpublished treatise *Discourses on Government* (*Seidan* 政談, ca. 1727), where he argued that the high cost of urban living encouraged doctors to prescribe mild treatments that would maximize their profits rather than harsher drugs that would bring about more effective cures. He therefore suggested that the *bakufu* should sponsor a medical school and send its graduates out to the countryside, where they would not face the temptations to venality presented by life in the cities.[29] However, since Sorai's *Discourses on Government* remained unpublished throughout the Tokugawa period, Tōdō and Tōyō were probably unaware of the details of these arguments. Instead, they based their notions of the ideal social context for the practice of medicine on the *Rituals of Zhou* (*Zhouli* 周禮), which had described a formal system of medical offices supposedly established by the Zhou government.

Tōdō argued that the medical system of the *Rituals of Zhou* revealed that medicine had long suffered from a confusion among categories of medical practice that should have been distinct. According to this scheme, there had been four branches of medicine corresponding to four classes of practitioner—physicians (*shitsu-i* 疾醫), dieticians (*shoku-i* 食醫), surgeons (*yō-i* 瘍醫), and veterinarians (*jū-i* 獸醫)—while later periods had also seen the

---

27   Yoshimasu (1759) 1918a, 448; cf. Ogyū (1717) 1973a, 28, 206; (1717) 1973b, 150, 244. For other examples of Tōdō's criticisms of "Principle," see Yoshimasu (1764) 1918b, 246–247; (1800) 1918e, 503–504; (1814) 1918f, 44, 45, 47.

28   Yamawaki Tōyō 1759, 1:6a. For discussion, see Yōrō 1996, 203. Yōrō suggests that a supposed distinction between nature and artifice in Sorai's political thought provided the basis for Tōyō's vision of the anatomical body as part of nature and thus as a possible object of knowledge. This provocative claim encounters three major difficulties: (1) it assumes the validity of Maruyama Masao's (1974) influential but controversial interpretation of Ogyū Sorai's "modernity"; (2) it imposes an anachronistic category of "nature" onto the ideas of eighteenth-century writers; (3) by positioning Tōyō's anatomical studies on a line of development running from Sorai to Sugita Genpaku rather than seeing them in the context of Tōyō's practical and polemical aims as an advocate of Ancient Formulas medicine, it neglects the role of philology in shaping Tōyō's observations and thus presents an exaggerated picture of his methodological empiricism.

29   Ogyū (1727) 1973c, 300, 390, 444.

development of yin-yang doctors (*in'yō-i* 陰陽醫) and Daoist doctors (*senka-i* 仙家醫). Tōdō deduced from the case histories recorded in the biography of the Western Han doctor Chunyu Yi 淳于意 that the ideas of yin-yang doctors had already by this period begun to displace those of true physicians, while later Chinese doctors such as Ge Hong 葛洪, Tao Hongjing 陶弘景, and Sun Simiao 孫思邈 had incorporated Daoist techniques for the cultivation of *qi* and for the production of elixirs to develop a distinctive tradition of Daoist medicine.[30] He concluded that no doctor had transmitted the ancient Way of physicians (*ko shitsu-i no michi* 古疾醫の道) since the time of Zhang Zhongjing, and that even the treatises of Tang dynasty authors included no more than a few genuinely ancient formulas.[31]

Tōdō and Tōyō developed their image of the ideal doctor as simultaneously a philologist and a practitioner by ascribing this dual identity to Zhang Zhongjing, about whom the scarcity of surviving biographical information allowed ample scope for imaginative reconstruction. The original preface to Zhongjing's *Treatise on Cold Damage Disorders* (*Shanghan lun* 傷寒論) stated that he had "diligently sought out the ancient precepts, widely gathering numerous formulas" 勤求古訓，博採眾方, and Tōdō and Tōyō deduced from this statement that Zhongjing's formulas had already been "ancient" when he had recorded them and that Zhongjing had preserved and transmitted these formulas in precisely the same way that Tōdō and Tōyō sought to preserve and transmit them during their own time. Tōyō declared that "Zhongjing followed the ancient precepts, preserving the methods and transmitting the art; ever since the death of Zhongjing, only Wang Tao in his *Medical Secrets from the Royal Library* 'transmitted and did not create.'"[32] Tōdō agreed with this evaluation of Zhongjing's achievement, stating that Zhongjing was "a transmitter of formulas, not a creator of formulas."[33] In adapting Sorai's methods and combining textual and empirical investigations in their efforts to recover the ancient art of medicine, Tōdō and Tōyō believed they were following the example of Zhang Zhongjing himself.

---

30   Yoshimasu (1814) 1918f, 44–47.

31   Yoshimasu (1759) 1918a, 451; (1769) 1918c, 2–3. For Tōyō's expression of a similar narrative of decline, see Yamawaki Tōyō 1759, 1:5b.

32   Yamawaki Tōyō 1751, 10b–11a.

33   Yoshimasu (1759) 1918a, 451; (1800) 1918e, 504, 512.

Anatomy and Philology in Yamawaki Tōyō's *Record of the Organs*

During his early medical studies, Yamawaki Tōyō had studied the descriptions of the body's organs in the orthodox medical classics *Basic Questions* (*Suwen* 素問), *Divine Pivot* (*Lingshu* 靈樞), and *Classic of Difficulties* (*Nanjing* 難經). It was Gotō Konzan who first suggested to Tōyō that dissection of human corpses might be the best way to learn the truth about the organs, but since this was prohibited, the best he could do was to conduct dissections on the corpses of otters (*kawauso* 獺), whose organs were thought to be similar. It was not until 1754 that Tōyō was given the opportunity to observe the dissection of an executed criminal's corpse, watching as the officially appointed "butcher" (*tosha* 屠者) cut open the body to reveal its contents.[34] Tōyō published his conclusions from these observations five years later in his *Record of the Organs* (*Zōshi* 蔵志, 1759), a book that helped stimulate the rapidly growing enthusiasm for anatomical knowledge among Japanese doctors during the following decades.

Given the importance of anatomy for the subsequent history of Japanese interest in European medicine, it is not surprising that historians have generally emphasized aspects of Tōyō's treatise that anticipated the later work of Sugita Genpaku 杉田玄白 (1733–1817) and other advocates of *rangaku* 蘭学 (Dutch Learning): the epistemological significance of visual observation, the role of European books as a stimulus to inquiry, or the use of illustrations as a way of representing knowledge to readers.[35] Yet as Yamada Keiji has pointed out, the tendency to view Tōyō's investigations retrospectively through their relationship to later Tokugawa anatomy risks distorting our understanding of Tōyō's intentions.[36] To understand the original significance of Tōyō's dissections, we need to consider more carefully how they were shaped by his practical aims and polemical purposes as an advocate of Ancient Formulas.

Tōyō's anatomical inquiries were motivated not simply by curiosity or by a desire to overturn received wisdom but by a practical concern to establish the universal human body—the target of Zhang Zhongjing's formulas—as a particular type of epistemic object, susceptible to investigation using the evidence provided by philology and direct observation. Seen from this perspective, Tōyō's anatomical treatise appears less as a precursor to Sugita Genpaku's *New Book of Anatomy* (*Kaitai shinsho* 解体新書, 1774) than as an extension of the

---

34   Yamawaki Tōyō 1759, 1:1a–3a. For a partial translation of this passage, see Fukuoka 2012, 35–36.

35   Fujikawa 1941, 404–409; Hattori 1978, 10; Johnston 1981; Okamoto 1988; Kuriyama 1992, 24–25; Yōrō 1996; Sakai 1997; Fukuoka 2012, 34–42; Aoki 2012, 71–75.

36   Yamada 1997.

project of evidential scholarship that Tōyō had begun several years previously in his edition of Wang Tao's *Medical Secrets from the Royal Library*.

This view of the body as a stable object knowable through evidential study was opposed to medical concepts of the variability of the body through time and space in the styles of medicine that had developed in China between the Song and the Ming dynasties and were popularized in Japan in the seventeenth century by the followers of Manase Dōsan 曲直瀬道三 (1507–1594).[37] This variability provided a justification for the cultivated intuition and complex doctrines that elite Chinese and Japanese doctors had claimed were necessary to devise therapeutic strategies best suited to the unique circumstances of individual patients. Several years before he carried out his dissections, Tōyō had already begun to develop arguments against this view, asserting that Zhongjing's formulas remained a reliable guide to therapy precisely because the human body was the same in all times and places:

> Who knows the causes of change and alteration? Is it not natural that restoring antiquity should be difficult? Nevertheless, the seven apertures have the same form, and the nine organs are all present. Light clothes in summer and heavy clothes in winter; becoming drunk with wine, becoming sated with meat. How can the human body change? Our nourishment and clothing do not alter, so why would our illnesses be different? The uses of drugs and stone needles can also be known from this. This is why our art is easy to know.[38]

Tōyō's excitement upon seeing Western anatomical treatises likewise derived not so much from their representational accuracy as from the fact that they demonstrated the universal nature of the human body: "The organs of [the sage ruler] Yao, the organs of [the tyrant ruler] Jie, and the organs of foreigners are all similar ... through a thousand ages they do not change, and across different regions they do not differ."[39] The stability of the human body across different regions of space provided indirect support for Tōyō's more important

---

37   On the variability of the human body in the Chinese medical "geographic imagination,"
      see Hanson 2011. On the history of Tokugawa ideas about Sino-Japanese medical differ-
      ence, see Trambaiolo 2013.

38   Yamawaki Tōyō 1751, 3b. Tōyō made a similar point in a letter sent to Hattori Nankaku in
      the eighth month of 1752: "The nine organs and the seven emotions are the same in antiq-
      uity and in the present. Wearing heavy cloth in winter and light cloth in summer—what
      difference is there between [the ages of] Yao and Jie? The illnesses from which they suf-
      fered can also be known" (Yamawaki Tōyō 1759, 2:17a).

39   Yamawaki Tōyō 1759, 1:6a; cf. Fukuoka 2012, 38.

assumption that the characteristics of the human body were stable through time, since stability through time was a necessary condition for the possibility of developing a style of medicine based on ancient formulas.

One of the major contrasts between the *Record of the Organs* and later Japanese anatomical treatises was the extent to which Tōyō was concerned not only to describe what he saw but also to draw attention to what he did not see. Tōyō complained that doctors who followed the *Basic Questions* and *Canon of Difficulties* were at risk of "clinging to names and losing the facts," contrasting Zhang Zhongjing's precise use of language with the vague and inaccurate terms for disease found in later medical treatises and arguing that the problem had arisen due to the progressive proliferation of empty language that failed to correspond to genuine aspects of reality.[40] As medical language had become more elaborate, it had gradually displaced the simpler but more accurate understanding of the body that had served as the basis of medicine in antiquity and that Tōyō hoped to restore through the careful use of evidence derived from philological study and direct observation. Rather than seeking to establish visual observation as the ultimate criterion for anatomical understanding, Tōyō made use of his observations as part of a broader polemical strategy to support the medical ideas and practices he attributed to Zhang Zhongjing and to undermine the medical orthodoxy based on the *Basic Questions*, *Numinous Pivot*, and *Canon of Difficulties*.

Tōyō's argument that the small and large intestines should be regarded not as two distinct organs but rather as a single continuous organ running from the stomach to the anus provides one of the clearest illustrations of how Tōyō's aims and methods in the *Record of the Organs* differed from those of later Tokugawa anatomists. Tōyō did not merely claim that he was unable to distinguish between small and large intestines; rather, he regarded the absence of distinct small and large intestines as a positive finding, on the same level as his observation that there were no channels for the flow of *qi* (*keiraku* 經絡) in the arms and legs, and his argument for this conclusion depended on his textual studies just as much as on his anatomical observations.[41] In a range of ancient texts, including the *Book of Documents* (*Shangshu* 尚書), the *Liezi* 列子, and the *Treatise on Cold Damage Disorders* itself, the intestines were mentioned only as a single organ; just as importantly, counting the intestines as a single organ meant that the total number of organs would correspond neatly to the "nine organs" mentioned in the *Rituals of Zhou*. Tōyō concluded that the distinction between the large and small intestines was one of the many empty

40   Yamawaki Tōyō 1759, 1:2b, 1:22b.
41   Yamawaki Tōyō 1759, 1:4b–5a.

concepts that had entered later medical discourse through the influence of yin-yang and Daoist ideas.[42] Later Tokugawa anatomists had fewer difficulties in observing the distinction between the small and large intestines, in part because they were able to build on the experience of earlier dissections and could make more effective use of European anatomical treatises, but also because they lacked Tōyō's characteristic commitment to the integration of philological and observational evidence.[43]

Many of Tōyō's contemporaries were reluctant to accept Tōyō's assumptions about the status of the human body as an object of knowledge. His *Record of the Organs* encountered skepticism not only among traditionally minded doctors who felt Tōyō had failed to understand the nature of the organs in classical medical theory but also among other Ancient Formulas doctors who felt that medical knowledge ought to concern itself only with the relationship between diseases and therapies and that Tōyō's anatomical investigations offered no more than a distraction.

Sano Yasusada 佐野安貞 attacked Tōyō from an orthodox perspective in his *Refutation of the "Record of the Organs" (Hi zōshi* 非蔵志, 1760), claiming that whatever philological objections might be raised against the received text of the *Basic Questions*, its medical doctrines derived from an authentic transmission of the doctrines of the Yellow Emperor himself.[44] Sano did not deny the value of knowing the forms and positions of the organs, but he claimed that Tōyō's attempts to understand them through dissection had ignored the crucial distinction between organs that were simply physical forms (*keizō* 形蔵) and organs that were vital functioning entities (*shinzō* 神蔵); in order to understand the latter, the evidence of visual observation was inferior to the sorts of learning that could be obtained from the *Yellow Emperor's Inner Canon* (*Huangdi neijing* 黄帝内經).[45] The scholar Hayashi Kōan 林厚庵 wrote in his preface to the *Refutation of the "Record of the Organs"* that "[Sorai's followers] proclaim that ritual, music, punishments, and government are the Way. They do not know that nature, the Way, and cultivation derive from Heaven. It is therefore only natural that they should also regard a deceased shell

---

42   Yamawaki Tōyō 1759, 1:2a–b, 1:5b. As Yamada Keiji has pointed out, this group of texts represented a highly selective reading of the available textual sources and commentaries: for a detailed analysis, see Yamada 1997, 477–479. For a comparison of Tōyō's description of the intestines with those found in other anatomical treatises popular in mid-eighteenth-century Japan, see Yōrō 1996, 205–218.

43   On the history of anatomical studies between Tōyō's *Record of the Organs* (1759) and Sugita Genpaku's *New Book of Anatomy* (1774), see Macé 1995; Yōrō 1996; Aoki 2012, 76–79.

44   Sano 1760, 1a–b.

45   Sano 1760, 2a, 3b–4a; cf. Fukuoka 2012, 38.

and decaying intestines as the Way."[46] In making these criticisms, Sano and Hayashi recognized that just as Sorai had insisted that moral and political discourse should refer to the concrete "forms" (*katachi/kei* 形) of social and political institutions, Tōyō's anatomical investigations were premised on the idea that medical discourse should refer to the concrete forms of the human body.[47]

Yoshimasu Tōdō was more skeptical than Tōyō about the value of inquiring into the physical structure of the organs: although he admitted that the *Rituals of Zhou* had stated that familiarity with the organs formed part of a doctor's responsibilities, he argued that references to the organs in the *Treatise on Cold Damage Disorders* were not part of Zhongjing's original text but had been added by later writers.[48] Two years after the publication of the *Record of the Organs*, Tōdō's disciple Tanaka Hidenobu 田中榮信 wrote a brief criticism of Tōyō's treatise from the perspective of this narrow conception of the scope of medical knowledge as strictly concerned with therapy.[49] Tanaka admired Tōyō's goal of restoring the medical profession of the Zhou and the medical techniques of the Han, but he argued that by focusing on internal bodily structures that had no relevance to the needling, moxa, and drug therapies that doctors used in practice, from a true physician's point of view Tōyō's descriptions of the organs ultimately resulted in precisely the same sort of empty discourse divorced from practice that Tōyō himself had sought to avoid.

Philology and Empiricism in Yoshimasu Tōdō's Pharmacology

Yoshimasu Tōdō was notorious for his use of aggressive sweating, purging, and vomiting therapies, which he justified by quoting a passage in the *Book of Documents*: "If the medicine is not *menken*, the disease will not be cured" 若藥弗瞑眩、厥疾弗瘳.[50] The usage of the term *menken* in its original context was metaphorical and its literal meaning unclear, but it apparently alluded to harsh

---

46   Sano 1760, preface by Hayashi Kōan, 1a.

47   Ogyū Sorai himself had accepted the conventional understanding of the organs as functional entities rather than physical forms, approving of Ujita Un'an's argument that "the *zō* and *fu* organs cannot be seen through dissection." See Ujita 1681, 4:2b–7b; Ogyū (1767) 1995, 27a.

48   Yoshimasu (1759) 1918a, 446.

49   Tanaka (1783) 1846, 40a–b.

50   Yoshimasu (1785) 1918d, 179–180. The earliest identified use of the term *menken* in Tokugawa medical discourse appears in a letter written by Yamawaki Tōyō in 1752 and published seven years later in an appendix to his *Record of the Organs*. Tōyō's use of the term at this early date may have been influenced by discussions with Tōdō, but Tōyō him-

effects such as dizziness or fainting. Later Chinese medical writers had occasionally alluded to this passage, but they had never made *menken* a central term for understanding the action of medicines in general; in particular, Zhang Zhongjing never made use of the term in any of his surviving writings. Nevertheless, Tōdō claimed to find the concept implicit in certain passages of the *Treatise on Cold Damage Disorders* and asserted that it was the key to understanding Zhang Zhongjing's approach to therapy.

Tōdō's therapies could sometimes be harsh enough to bring his patients to the brink of death, and he readily admitted that the *menken* of his drugs could be so extreme as to give the appearance that his patients had died from consuming them.[51] However, Tōdō argued that even if his patients passed away after receiving his treatment, he could have no regrets, since their fate was determined not by his remedies but by the command of Heaven (*tenmei* 天命).[52] Tōdō found support for this doctrine in Sima Qian's biography of the legendary doctor Bian Que 扁鵲, who had supposedly remarked after his successful treatment of the apparently deceased crown prince of Guo 虢, "I am not able to bring the dead to life: this man was meant to live, and I merely caused him to arise."[53] Tōdō's critics were quick to point out the logical flaws and moral dangers of these arguments.[54] However, even these opponents regarded the study of ancient Chinese texts as an essential source of evidence to be used in arriving at the correct doctrine: Hata Kōzan 畑黄山 (1720–1804), for example, pointed out that historical evidence such as the *Rituals of Zhou*'s stipulation that doctors' salaries should be determined according to their patients' rates of survival contradicted Tōdō's claim that the doctors of antiquity did not concern themselves with life and death.[55] Despite their divergent ideas about medicine and about the social roles of doctors, even doctors who opposed Tōdō had come to share his assumption that some important medical questions could only be settled by making reference to ancient texts beyond those of the medical canon itself.

This assumption formed the basis of Tōdō's approach to pharmacology, which employed a combination of textual research and direct observation similar to that of Yamawaki Tōyō in his anatomical studies. Earlier Chinese and

---

self regarded the concept as too simplistic to serve as an adequate guide to the complexities of medical therapy: see Yamawaki Tōyō 1759, 1:5b, 1:26a, 2:9a.

51   Yoshimasu (1769) 1918c, 9–12, 19–20.

52   Yoshimasu (1759) 1918a, 444–445.

53   Yoshimasu (1769) 1918c, 3.

54   Aoki 2012, 85–87.

55   Hata 1762, 7a.

Japanese treatises on the properties of drugs had generally adhered to the conventions of the genre of materia medica (Ch. *bencao*, J. *honzō* 本草), at the apogee of which stood Li Shizhen's *Systematic Materia Medica (Bencao gangmu* 本草綱目, 1596).[56] This genre had traditionally incorporated learning of a highly heterogeneous nature, combining pharmacological knowledge about the therapeutic properties of drugs with encyclopedic description of the many varieties of plant, animal, and mineral products. A number of Japanese scholars in the late seventeenth and early eighteenth centuries were working to develop a distinctive Japanese variant of this tradition, gradually distancing *honzōgaku* 本草学 (material medica) from its original association with medicine and establishing it as a broader field of natural historical knowledge.[57] These developments in Tokugawa *honzōgaku* opened up new possibilities for thinking about pharmacology itself as a field of knowledge distinct from broader investigations into the natural world. Kagawa Shūan had begun to explore these possibilities in his *Ippondō's Selected Pharmaceuticals (Ippondō yakusen* 一本堂藥選, 1731–1738), and Yoshimasu Tōdō developed his own distinctive account of pharmacology in his *Pharmacological Demonstrations (Yakuchō* 藥徵, 1785).

In this treatise, Tōdō sought to provide a set of foundations for pharmacological knowledge independent of the materia medica tradition. Tōdō spent three decades revising this treatise, and throughout his lifetime he refused to have it published; it was only after his son and heir Yoshimasu Nangai 吉益南涯 arranged for its publication in 1785 that it became established as one of Tōdō's most influential works.[58] Tōdō's pharmacological investigations were based on the premise that although the materia medica tradition included valuable knowledge that should not be discarded, it was compromised not only by its indiscriminate mixture of correct and incorrect doctrines but also by its failure to distinguish between the types of knowledge appropriate to physicians (*shitsu-i* 疾醫) and those appropriate to dieticians (*shoku-i* 食醫).[59] He argued that the distinction in the materia medica between drugs "with poison" (*yūdoku* 有毒) and drugs "without poison" (*mudoku* 無毒) followed from this basic confusion and exemplified the problem with the materia medica for the aspiring physician. Tōdō regarded "poison" as an essential char-

---

56   Nappi 2009.

57   Yamada 1995; Marcon 2007; Sugimoto 2011; Fukuoka 2012.

58   Ōtsuka 1985, 26–27. Regarding Yoshimasu Tōdō's reluctance to publish this book, see Yoshimasu Nangai's colophon to Yoshimasu (1785) 1918d, 242.

59   Yoshimasu (1759) 1918a, 449; (1785) 1918d, 139–140, 154.

acter of all drugs that was fundamental to their ability to expel disease.[60] He thus claimed that the distinction between drugs with and without poison was a consequence of the fact that the materia medica had not been written from a perspective appropriate to physicians but had been assembled from a variety of dietetic, yin-yang, and Daoist sources.[61] Compiling a pharmacological treatise to meet the needs of true physicians thus demanded an independent set of foundations for pharmacology based on a combination of philological study of the *Treatise on Cold Damage Disorders* with direct practical experience.

The treatises of Zhang Zhongjing had presented the efficacy of drugs not as isolated substances but only as components of formulas; to reconstruct Zhongjing's implicit understanding of the medicinal properties of individual drugs, Tōdō therefore used a method that he referred to as "examination of the evidence" (*kōchō* 考徵). For each drug, he identified all the formulas in Zhongjing's treatise that included that drug, and by comparing the lists of symptoms corresponding to each of these formulas, he deduced the specific healing properties of individual drugs from the set of symptoms that were listed under all the formulas in which that drug occurred and absent from the formulas in which the drug did not occur.[62] In some cases, Tōdō made reference to textual parallels in the writings of Tang dynasty doctors such as Sun Simiao and Wang Tao, using these parallels to emend passages of Zhang Zhongjing's treatise for which he suspected the received text had become corrupted in transmission.[63] Despite such complications, Tōdō was confident that this method would provide more precise knowledge of the nature of drugs, and that this would in turn lead to better understanding of the formulas themselves.[64]

To support his conclusions concerning the effects of individual drugs, Tōdō cited cases from his own practical experience that contradicted the received ideas of the materia medica tradition. He used this evidence to show that gypsum (*sekkō* 石膏) should not be regarded as a harsh drug but could be effectively prescribed over an extended period, that *Bupleurum* root (*saiko* 柴胡) was useful for treating periodic fevers (*gyakushitsu* 瘧疾) only in cases when these were accompanied by painful swelling around the chest and sides, that *Pinellia* tuber (*hange* 半夏) could be safely administered during pregnancy, that ginseng should be used for clearing dense accumulations below the heart

60   Yoshimasu (1785) 1918d, 146; cf. Kagawa 1734, *hanrei* 3b.

61   Yoshimasu (1785) 1918d, 241.

62   Yoshimasu (1785) 1918d, 153.

63   Yoshimasu (1785) 1918d, 144, 202.

64   Yoshimasu (1759) 1918a, 451.

(*shinge hikō* 心下痞硬) rather than as a general-purpose supplementation drug (*hoyaku* 補藥), and that "warming" drugs were not necessarily the most effective treatment for patients suffering from coldness in their extremities.[65] Tōdō's references to clinical experience as evidence for drug efficacy were much less systematic than his careful deductions from the text of the *Treatise on Cold Damage Disorders*, and he seems to have regarded his textual research and his clinical experiences as mutually validating rather than as potentially conflicting sources of evidence. Tōdō's *Pharmacological Demonstrations*, like Tōyō's *Record of the Organs*, represented an attempt to demonstrate that the conclusions to be drawn from textual sources were identical to those that would be drawn from direct observation and practical experience.

Conclusion

Although the conclusions of Tōdō's and Tōyō's medical investigations did not depend in any substantive way on Sorai's political or philosophical doctrines, their epistemic affinities ran deeper than the mere appropriation of Sorai's rhetoric. These affinities were based on the analogous ways in which Sorai and Tōdō and Tōyō construed the relationship between contemporary knowledge, the objects of that knowledge, and historical traditions of learned discourse. This structural parallel between Sorai's social thought and Tōdō's and Tōyō's medical ideas suggests that we should see the latter, not as an expression of a straightforward empiricism in which the authority of texts was to be replaced by that of experience, but as one in which experience was to be used strategically in the affirmation, rejection, and reinterpretation of textual evidence that had itself become open to reevaluation through the methods of philological scholarship.

With the declining influence of Sorai's ideas in the second half of the eighteenth century, fewer and fewer doctors felt the same sense of a necessary connection between philological and empirical investigation that Tōdō and Tōyō had felt during the century's middle decades, and within a few years of their deaths the notion that the conclusions of philology would correspond precisely to those of practical investigations began to seem increasingly implausible. Tōyō's son and heir Yamawaki Tōmon 山脇東門 (1736–1782) wrote disparagingly of Yoshimasu Tōdō as a doctor who had "followed after the epigones of Sorai and acquired a smattering of knowledge about ancient phraseology," apparently overlooking the fact that the same might have been said about his

---

65   Yoshimasu (1785) 1918d, 145–146, 177, 189, 202, 217.

own father.[66] Doctors who had initially been enthusiastic about Ancient Formulas began to doubt that Zhang Zhongjing's formulas would offer a sufficiently broad range of therapies to cure the diseases that Japanese doctors encountered in practice.[67] The publication of Sugita Genpaku's *New Book of Anatomy* (1774) made Yamawaki Tōyō's anatomical investigations seem crude, not only by surpassing them in detail but also by introducing a new set of criteria that established anatomy as a form of visual knowledge.[68] Many subsequent doctors appropriated and extended various aspects of Tōdō's and Tōyō's legacy: philological studies of medical texts continued to attract the efforts of scholarly doctors into the final years of the Tokugawa period; use of and experimentation with Zhang Zhongjing's formulas were even more widespread; and Yoshimasu Tōdō is widely admired by contemporary *kanpō* practitioners even today. However, their particular conception of the nature of medical knowledge and evidence could not be passed on intact to the generations that followed them: it was too closely tied to the intellectual and social conditions of their own time.

References

Anzai Yasuchika 安西安周 1943. *Nihon jui kenkyū* 日本儒医研究 [Research on Confucian doctors in Japan]. Tokyo: Ryūginsha.

Aoki Toshiyuki 青木歳幸 2012. *Edo jidai no igaku: meiitachi no 300 nen* 江戸時代の医学：名医たちの三〇〇年 [The medical learning of the Edo period: Three hundred years of famous doctors]. Tokyo: Yoshikawa kōbunkan.

Bitō Masahide 尾藤正英 2013. *Ogyū Sorai "Seidan"* 荻生徂徠「政談」 [Ogyū Sorai's *Discourses on government*]. Tokyo: Kōdansha.

Elman, Benjamin A. 2001. *From Philosophy to Philology: Intellectual and Social Aspects of Change in Late Imperial China*. 2nd rev. ed. Los Angeles: UCLA Asian Pacific Monograph Series.

Flueckiger, Peter 2011. *Imagining Harmony: Poetry, Empathy, and Community in Mid-Tokugawa Confucianism and Nativism*. Stanford, CA: Stanford University Press.

Fujikawa Yū 富士川游 1941. *Nihon igaku shi* 日本医学史 [History of medical learning in Japan]. Tokyo: Nisshin shoin.

Fukuoka, Maki 2012. *The Premise of Fidelity: Science, Visuality and Representing the Real in Tokugawa Japan*. Stanford, CA: Stanford University Press.

---

66   Yamawaki Tōmon (n.d.) 1924, 1.

67   For an example, see the remarks by Kamei Nanmei quoted in Yoshida 1999, 10–11.

68   Kuriyama 1992; Yōrō 1996; Fukuoka 2012, 39–42.

Gotō Konzan 後藤艮山 (n.d.) 1971. *Shisetsu hikki* 師説筆記 [Written transcription of the teacher's doctrines]. Reprinted in *Nihon shisō taikei* 日本思想大系, vol. 63, edited by Ōtsuka Keisetsu 大塚敬節. Tokyo: Iwanami shoten.

Hanson, Marta 2011. *Speaking of Epidemics in Chinese Medicine: Disease and the Geographic Imagination in Late Imperial China.* London: RoutledgeCurzon.

Hata Kōzan 畑黄山 1762. *Seki idan* 斥医断 [Rebuttal of *Judgments on medicine*].

Hattori Toshirō 服部敏郎 1978. *Edo jidai igakushi no kenkyū* 江戸時代医学史の研究 [Research on the history of medical learning in the Edo period]. Tokyo: Yoshikawa kōbunkan.

Johnston, William D. 1981. "Jūhasseiki Nihon no igaku ni okeru kagaku kakumei: Ranpō no hatten no tame no shisōteki na zentei" 十八世紀日本の医学における科学革命：蘭方の発展のための思想的な前提 [A scientific revolution in eighteenth-century medicine: Intellectual preconditions for the development of Dutch Learning]. *Nihon ishigaku zasshi* 27, 1: 6–20; 27, 2: 131–156.

Kagawa Shūan 香川修庵 1734. *Ippondō yakusen* 一本堂薬選 [Ippondō's selected pharmaceuticals].

——— 1744. *Iji setsuyaku* 医事説約 [Concise explanation of medical matters].

Kamei Nanmei 亀井南冥 1764. *Ōō yokyō* 泱泱余響 [Lingering reverberations of vastness].

Kasaya Kazuhiko 笠谷和比古 2011. "Joron: Jūhasseiki Nihon no 'chi'-teki kakumei" 序論：十八世紀日本の「知」的革命 [Preface: The revolution in "knowledge" in eighteenth-century Japan], in Kasaya Kazuhiko, ed., *Jūhasseiki Nihon no bunka jōkyō to kokusai kankyō* 一八世紀日本の文化状況と国際環境. Kyoto: Shibunkaku shuppan, 3–29.

Kornicki, Peter 1998. *The Book in Japan: A Cultural History from the Beginnings to the Nineteenth Century.* Leiden: E. J. Brill.

Kosoto Hiroshi 小曽戸洋 1999. *Kanpō no rekishi: Chūgoku, Nihon no dentō igaku* 漢方の歴史：中国、日本の伝統医学 [The history of *kanpō*: The traditional medicine of China and Japan]. Tokyo: Taishūkan shoten.

Kure Shūzō 呉秀三 1918. "Yoshimasu Tōdō sensei" 吉益東洞先生 [Master Yoshimasu Tōdō], in Kure Shūzō 呉秀三 and Fujikawa Yū 富士川游, eds., *Tōdō zenshū*. Tokyo: Tohōdō shoten.

Kuriyama, Shigehisa 1992. "Between Mind and Eye: Japanese Anatomy in the Eighteenth Century," in Charles Lesley and Allan Young, eds., *Paths to Asian Medical Knowledge.* Berkeley: University of California Press, 21–43.

Lan Hongyue 藍弘岳 2007. "Ogyū Sorai no shisō keisei ni okeru igaku to heigaku: *Sorai sensei igen* to *Sonshi kokujikai* wo chūshin ni" 荻生徂徠の思想形成における医学と兵学：『徂徠先生医言』と『孫子国字解』を中心に [Medical learning and military learning in the intellectual formation of Ogyū Sorai: With special attention to *Master Sorai's medical sayings* and *Kana explanations of Sunzi*], *Nihon shisōshigaku* 39: 75–94.

Macé, Mieko 1995. "Dissection, Blood-Letting and Medicine as per Yamawaki Tōmon and Ogino Gengai," in Hashimoto Keizō, Catherine Jami, and Lowell Skar, eds., *East Asian Science: Tradition and Beyond; Papers from the Seventh International Conference on the History of Science in East Asia, Kyoto, 2–7 August 1993*. Osaka: Kansai University Press, 351–357.

——— 1997. "La médecine de Hoashi Banri (1778–1852): Recherche d'une médecine universelle par un naturaliste encyclopédiste de la première moitié du XIXe siècle," in J. Pigeot and H. O. Rotermund, eds., *La vase de Béryl: Études sur le Japon et la Chine en hommage à Bernard Frank*. Arles: Éditions Philippe Picquier, 405–415.

Machi Senjurō 町泉寿郎 1998a. "Kagawa Shūan no 'ju-i ippon' no ju ni tsuite: *Daigakusō* wo chūshin to shite" 香川修庵の「儒医一本」の儒について：『大学叢』を中心として [On the Confucianism in Kagawa Shūan's "Confucianism and medicine have a single root": With special attention to *Daigakusō*], *Nihon ishigaku zasshi* 44, 1: 49–72.

——— 1998b. "Yamawaki Tōyō to Sorai gakuha: *Waitai miyao fang* honkoku wo megutte" 山脇東洋と徂徠学派：『外台秘要方』翻刻をめぐって [Yamawaki Tōyō and the Sorai school: On the reprinting of *Medical secrets from the Royal Library*], *Nihon Chūgokugaku kaihō* 50: 233–47.

Marcon, Federico 2007. "The Names of Nature: The Development of Natural History in Japan, 1600–1900." Ph.D. diss., Columbia University.

Maruyama Masao 1974. *Studies in the Intellectual History of Tokugawa Japan*, translated by Mikiso Hane. Princeton, NJ: Princeton University Press.

Nagatomi Dokushōan 永富独嘯庵 (1764) 1807. *Man'yū zakki* 漫遊雑記 [Miscellaneous notes while roaming at leisure].

Najita, Tetsuo 1998. *Tokugawa Political Writings.* Cambridge: Cambridge University Press.

Nakamura Shunsaku 中村春作 1996. "Sorai wa dō 'yomareta' ka?" 徂徠はどう「読まれ」たか [How was Sorai "read"?], *Edo no shisō* 5: 29–47.

Nappi, Carla 2009. *The Monkey and the Inkpot: Natural History and Its Transformations in Early Modern China.* Cambridge, MA: Harvard University Press.

Ogyū Sorai 荻生徂徠 (1717) 1973a. *Bendō* 弁道 [Disputing the Way]. Reprinted in *Nihon shisō taikei* 日本思想大系, vol. 36, edited by Yoshikawa Kōjirō 吉川幸次郎. Tokyo: Iwanami shoten.

——— (1717) 1973b. *Benmei* 弁名 [Disputing names]. Reprinted in *Nihon shisō taikei* 日本思想大系, vol. 36, edited by Yoshikawa Kōjirō 吉川幸次郎. Tokyo: Iwanami shoten.

——— (1727) 1973c. *Seidan* 政談 [Discourses on government]. Reprinted in *Nihon shisō taikei* 日本思想大系, vol. 36, edited by Yoshikawa Kōjirō 吉川幸次郎. Tokyo: Iwanami shoten.

———— (1767) 1995. *Sorai sensei igen* 徂徠先生医言 [Master Sorai's sayings on medicine]. Reprinted in *Rinshō kanpō shohō kaisetsu* 臨床漢方処方解説. Osaka: Oriento shuppansha.

Okamoto Takashi 岡本喬 1988. *Kaibō kotohajime: Yamawaki Tōyō no hito to shisō* 解剖事始め：山脇東洋の人と思想 [The beginnings of anatomy: The life and thought of Yamawaki Tōyō]. Tokyo: Dōseisha.

Ōtsuka Keisetsu 大塚敬節 1985. "Yoshimasu Tōdō" 吉益東洞, in Ōtsuka Keisetsu, ed., *Kinsei kanpō igakusho shūsei* 近世漢方医学書集成, vol. 10. Tokyo: Meicho shuppan, 7–38.

Rai Kiichi 頼祺一 1993. "Kinseijin ni totte no gakumon to jissen" 近世人によっての学問と実践 [Early modern people's views of putting learning into practice], in Rai Kiichi, ed., *Nihon no kinsei: Jugaku, kokugaku, yōgaku* 日本の近世：儒学，国学，洋学. Tokyo: Chūō kōronsha, 7–34.

Rubinger, Richard 2007. *Popular Literacy in Early Modern Japan.* Honolulu: University of Hawai'i Press.

Sakai Shizu 酒井シヅ 1997. "Jūshichi, jūhachi seiki no nihonjin no shintaikan" 一七、一八世紀の日本人の身体観 [Views of the body among Japanese people of the seventeenth and eighteenth centuries], in Yamada Keiji 山田慶児 and Kuriyama Shigehisa 栗山茂久, eds., *Rekishi no naka no yamai to igaku* 歴史の中の病と医学. Kyoto: Shibunkaku, 431–455.

Sano Yasusada 佐野安貞 1760. *Hi zōshi* 非蔵志 [Refutation of the *Record of the Organs*].

Sugimoto, Masayoshi, and David L. Swain 1978. *Science and Culture in Traditional Japan.* Cambridge, MA: MIT Press.

Sugimoto Tsutomu 杉本つとむ 2011. *Nihon honzōgaku no sekai: Shizen, iyaku, minzoku goi no tankyū* 日本本草学の世界: 自然、医薬、民俗語彙の探究 [The world of Japanese materia medica studies: Investigations of nature, medicines, and vernacular vocabulary]. Tokyo: Yasaka shobō.

Tanaka Hidenobu 田中栄信 (1783) 1846. *Ben seki idan* 辨斥医断 [Disputing the *Rebuttal of the Judgment on Medicine*].

Tateno Masami 館野正美 2004. *Yoshimasu Tōdō "Kosho igen" no kenkyū: Sono shoshi to igaku shisō* 吉益東洞『古書医言』の研究：その書誌と医学思想 [Research on Yoshimasu Tōdō's *Medical sayings from ancient books*: Bibliography and medical ideas]. Tokyo: Kyūko shoin.

Terasawa Katsutoshi 寺澤捷年 2012. *Yoshimasu Tōdō no kenkyū: Nihon kanpō sōzō no shisō* 吉益東洞の研究：日本漢方創造の思想 [Research on Yoshimasu Tōdō: The ideas that created Japanese *kanpō*]. Tokyo: Iwanami shoten.

Trambaiolo, Daniel 2013. "Native and Foreign in Tokugawa Medicine," *Journal of Japanese Studies* 39, 2: 299–324.

———— 2014a. "Diplomatic Journeys and Medical Brush Talks: Eighteenth-Century Dialogues between Korean and Japanese Medicine," in Ofer Gal and Yi Zheng, eds.,

Motion and Knowledge in the Changing Early Modern World: Orbits, Routes and Vessels. Dordrecht: Springer Verlag, 93–113.

——— 2014b. "The Languages of Medical Knowledge in Tokugawa Japan," in Benjamin Elman, ed. *Rethinking East Asian Languages, Vernaculars, and Literacies, 1000–1919.* Leiden: E. J. Brill, 147–168.

Tucker, John A. 2006. *Ogyū Sorai's Philosophical Masterworks: The "Bendō" and "Benmei."* Honolulu: University of Hawai'i Press.

Ujita Un'an 宇治田雲南 1681. *Igaku bengai* 医学辨害 [Discriminating the harms of medicine].

Yamada Keiji 山田慶児, ed. 1995. *Higashi Ajia no honzō to hakubutsugaku no sekai* 東アジアの本草と博物学の世界 [The worlds of East Asian materia medica and natural history]. Kyoto: Shibunkaku shuppan.

——— 1997. "Igaku ni oite kogaku ha nan de atta ka: Yamawaki Tōyō no kaibōgaku to shokugyō oyobi gakumon to shite no i no jiritsu" 医学において古学はなんであったか：山脇東洋の解剖学と職業および学問としての医の自立 [What was ancient learning in medicine? The independence of medicine as an occupation and as a scholarly discipline in Yamawaki Tōyō's anatomical learning], in Yamada Keiji 山田慶児 and Kuriyama Shigehisa 栗山茂久, eds., *Rekishi no naka no yamai to igaku* 歴史の中の病と医学. Kyoto: Shibunkaku shuppan, 457–487.

——— 2006. "Hankagaku to shite no kohōha igaku" 反科学としての古方派医学 [Ancient Formulas medicine as antiscience], *Shisō* 985, 5: 26–65.

Yamawaki Tōmon 山脇東門 (n.d.) 1924. *Tōmon zuihitsu* 東門随筆 [Tōmon's miscellaneous writings]. Reprinted in Fujikawa Yū 富士川游, ed., *Kyōrin sōsho* 杏林叢書, vol. 3. Tohōdō shoten.

Yamawaki Tōyō 山脇東洋 1751. *Yōjuin isoku* 養寿院医則 [Yōjuin's medical principles]. Kyoto: Hayashi Gonbē and Hayashi Yoshibē.

——— 1759. *Zōshi* 蔵志 [Record of the organs].

——— (n.d.) 1979. *Tōyō rakugo* 東洋洛語 [Tōyō's words in the capital]. Reprinted in Ōtsuka Keisetsu 大塚敬節, ed., *Kinsei kanpō igakusho shūsei* 近世漢方医学書集成, vol. 13. Tokyo: Meicho shuppan.

Yokota Fuyuhiko 横田冬彦 1998. "Kinsei sonraku shakai ni okeru 'chi' no mondai" 近世村落社会における＜知＞の問題 [The problem of "knowledge" in early modern village society], *Hisutoria* 159, 1–28.

Yōrō Takeshi 養老孟司 1996. "Edo no kaibōzu" 江戸の解剖図 [Anatomical diagrams of the Edo period], in Takashina Shūji 高階秀爾, ed., *Edo no naka no kindai: Akita ranga to* Kaitai shinsho 江戸のなかの近代：秋田蘭画と『解体新書』. Tokyo: Chikuma shobō, 189–228.

Yoshida Yōichi 吉田洋一 1999. "Kamei Nanmei no igaku shisō" 亀井南冥の医学思想 [The medical ideas of Kamei Nanmei], *Yōgaku* 8: 1–21.

Yoshikawa Kōjirō 1983. *Jinsai, Sorai, Norinaga: Three Classical Philologists of Mid-Tokugawa Japan*, translated by Kikuchi Yūji. Tokyo: Tōhō Gakkai.

Yoshimasu Tōdō 吉益東洞 (1759) 1918a. *Idan* 医断 [Judgments on medicine]. Reprinted in Kure Shūzō 呉秀三 and Fujikawa Yū 富士川游, eds., *Tōdō zenshū*. Tokyo: Tohōdō shoten.

——— (1764) 1918b. *Ruijuhō* 類聚方 [Classified formulas]. Reprinted in Kure Shūzō 呉秀三 and Fujikawa Yū 富士川游, eds., *Tōdō zenshū*. Tokyo: Tohōdō shoten.

——— (1769) 1918c. *Iji wakumon* 医事或問 [Answers to questions on medical matters]. Reprinted in Kure Shūzō 呉秀三 and Fujikawa Yū 富士川游, eds., *Tōdō zenshū*. Tokyo: Tohōdō shoten.

——— (1785) 1918d. *Yakuchō* 薬徴 [Pharmacological demonstrations]. Reprinted in Kure Shūzō 呉秀三 and Fujikawa Yū 富士川游, eds., *Tōdō zenshū*. Tokyo: Tohōdō shoten.

——— (1800) 1918e. *Tōdō sensei ikō* 東洞先生遺稿 [Master Tōdō's posthumous drafts]. Reprinted in Kure Shūzō 呉秀三 and Fujikawa Yū 富士川游, eds., *Tōdō zenshū*. Tokyo: Tohōdō shoten.

——— (1814) 1918f. *Kosho igen* 古書医言 [Medical sayings from ancient books]. Reprinted in Kure Shūzō 呉秀三 and Fujikawa Yū 富士川游, eds., *Tōdō zenshū*. Tokyo: Tohōdō shoten.

——— (1825) 1918g. *Tōdō ō isō* 東洞翁遺草 [Master Tōdō's posthumous writings]. Reprinted in Kure Shūzō 呉秀三 and Fujikawa Yū 富士川游, eds., *Tōdō zenshū*. Tokyo: Tohōdō shoten.

CHAPTER 5

The Reception of the Circulation Channels Theory in Japan (1500–1800)

Mathias Vigouroux

Today the channels theory is considered to be one of cornerstones of acupuncture therapy. Yet the picture prompted by contemporary acupuncture textbooks does not account for the profound transformation that this theory underwent since the first mention of *qi* and blood flowing inside channels in the *Guanzi* 管子 (compiled around the third century BCE).[1] Nor does it reveal anything about the contribution of China's neighboring countries to the recovery of original acupuncture texts lost or circulating only in a corrupted version in China. In the past decades, historians have paid attention to the evolution of the channels theory in China prior to the Qing dynasty (1368–1644) and its transmission to early modern Europe.[2] What remains relatively unexplored, however, is the circulation and appropriation of this theory within Asia, particularly why textbooks that had a key role in China in the dissemination of the channels theory had only a limited influence in Japan, whereas manuals of minor importance in China became central to Japanese acupuncturists.[3]

---

1   On the *Guanzi*, see Harper 1998, 77.

2   On the early development of the channels theory, see, e.g., Harper 1998; Unschuld 2003; Goldschmidt 2009; Yu 2007. See also Lo 2005; her analysis of the Dunhuang moxibustion charts reveals that a practice of cauterizing specific points on the body outside the network of channels did not cease to exist until the late Tang dynasty (618–908) despite the preeminence of the channels theory. On the transmission of acupuncture to Europe, see esp. Cook 2007, 2011; Barnes 2005; Unschuld 1995.

3   Machi (2008) tackles the question of the reception of Hua Shou's *Shisijing fahui* in Japan, focusing on the different editions circulating during the Tokugawa period. Nagano (2001a) offers a good introduction to acupuncture mannequins and charts. Mayanagi Makoto and Kosoto Hiroshi were the first to quantitatively identify the Chinese acupuncture classics transmitted to and reprinted in Japan during the medieval and early modern period; however, their works do not address the question of the reception of these classics. See Mayanagi and Tomobe 1992; Mayanagi 2001; Kosoto, Seki, and Kurihara 1990. Andrew Goble's most recent book (2011) on medicine in medieval Japan focuses exclusively on the new developments in pharmacopeia formulas in relation to their Japanese interpretations. He does not discuss how the new acupuncture texts published in Song China

By determining what Chinese textbooks were available to Japanese physicians and how they selected them and appropriated their content, this essay seeks to explore the early reception of the channels theory in Japan and the sort of challenges faced by Japanese physicians in assimilating it into their medical practice. I first review the reception of Chinese acupuncture in the classical and medieval periods, arguing that the turning point in Japan was the transmission of Hua Shou's 滑壽 *Shisijing fahui* 十四經發揮 (*Elucidation of the Fourteen Channels*, 1341) in the late medieval period. Although major Chinese medical books explaining the channels theory had been transmitted to Japan, knowledge about the channels was not diffused to a large number of Japanese physicians and was not yet applied to clinical practice prior to the introduction of Hua Shou's textbook. I analyze particularly the role that Manase Dōsan 曲直瀬道三 (1507–1594) played in the adoption of this textbook as the authoritative text on the channels theory. I also argue that the visual innovations in the representation of the course of the channels and the location of the acupuncture points on the body in the second half of the seventeenth century functioned as multimedia pedagogical tools to facilitate the acquisition of knowledge about the channels theory.

Acupuncture in Japan before 1500

Japanese medical books of the Heian (794–1185) and Kamakura (1185–1333) periods present a contrasting picture of acupuncture, which was first introduced in Japan around the sixth century via China and Korea.[4] They suggest that although Japanese physicians had access to all the basic Chinese medical treatises, acupuncture was rarely used in clinical practice compared to moxibustion and herbal remedies, and it was administrated essentially to treat ulcers, tumors, boils, and abscesses. In other words, acupuncture needles seem to have been employed merely as a kind of surgical tool. For instance, in the *Ishinpō* 醫心方 (*Formulas from the Heart of Medicine*), written in 984, the aristocrat

---

that represented a departure from previous periods were transmitted and appropriated in medieval Japan or how the works of the Japanese physicians reflected these changes.

4   The *Nihonshoki* 日本書紀 (*The Chronicles of Japan*, 720), for instance, records that in 562 CE, in the twenty-third year of Emperor Kimmei's 欽明 reign, Zhi Cong 智聰, originating from Wu 吳 in the southeastern part of China, brought to Japan 160 books, including several medical treatises. Only the title of one of them is mentioned: *Ming tang tu* 明堂圖 (*Numinous Hall Chart*). This is the first mention in Japan of a Chinese medical book related to acupuncture points.

physician Tanba no Yasuyori 丹波康頼 (912–995) makes few references to the pulse diagnosis and the channels theory.[5] Moxibustion is recommended in 361 cases, whereas acupuncture needles are mentioned in only 6 cases. Moreover, although Tanba refers to the nine needles first described in China in the *Huangdi neijing lingshu* 黃帝內經靈樞 (*The Yellow Emperor's Inner Classic: Divine Pivot*), but explicitly names only seven of them, there is no mention of a needle inserted at the location of an acupuncture point. They are always applied on the affected part of the body to treat abscesses and other purulent swellings.[6] This feature of the *Ishinpō*, however, was not specific to Japanese medicine. Chinese medical textbooks written during the Tang dynasty also privileged moxibustion therapy.[7] The relative underuse of acupuncture therapy during the Heian period was not specific to Japanese medicine and reflected therefore the state of acupuncture in China previous to the Song dynasty.

After the disintegration of the Han Empire (206 BCE–220 CE), the acupuncture classics circulated among a very limited number of physicians in China.[8] Only a few diagrams were available to help practitioners visualize the acupuncture points in the body.[9] Practitioners relied therefore principally on textual descriptions to locate them. However, over time, discrepancies appeared between treatises, and Chinese physicians became extremely cautious in using acupuncture in clinical practice. They privileged moxibustion instead; this therapy did not require complex knowledge, for moxa could be administered directly at the location of the ailment outside the framework of the acupuncture points.[10] Moxibustion was also a safer therapy. Immediate risks inherent to the practice of moxibustion were mostly limited to burns and blisters,

---

5   Only volume 22, on obstetrics 胎教篇, includes drawings representing the forbidden points during each stage of pregnancy (任婦脉圖月禁法). The original diagrams of chapter 12 in volume 2, titled *Numinous Hall Charts*, have been lost, so it is not possible to know whether they depicted both acupuncture channels and points or only acupuncture points.

6   Shinohara 1994, 109–110; Macé 1985, 454.

7   In the two volumes dedicated to acupuncture and moxibustion in Sun Simiao's 孫思邈 (581–682) *Beiji qianjin yaofang* 備急千金要方 (*Essential Recipes for Urgent Use Worth a Thousand Gold Pieces*, ca. 650–659), there are 560 references to moxibustion but only 90 to acupuncture. See Yu 2007, 323.

8   Goldschmidt 2009, 9.

9   The only diagrams still extant are the moxibustion charts in the Dunhuang collection reproduced in Lo 2005, 211–222.

10   For example, the Jin dynasty (265–316 CE) physician Chen Yanzhi 陳延之, quoted by Tanba no Yasuyori in the *Ishinpō* (1991, 247), explains that to practice acupuncture it was necessary to be trained by a teacher, whereas even ordinary persons could apply moxibustion.

whereas a needle wrongly inserted could cause bleeding, damage the tissues or the organs, and have even more dramatic consequences.[11] During the Tang dynasty, moxibustion even replaced decoction for people living in remote areas.[12]

A major turning point in the history of Chinese acupuncture was the publication in 1026 of Wang Weiyi's 王惟一 (987–1067) *Tongren yuxue zhenjiu tu jing* 銅人俞穴針灸圖經 (*Illustrated Classic of Acupuncture and Moxibustion Points on the Bronze Man*) and the casting one year later of two bronze figures (*tongren* 銅人) to model the acupuncture points. In the early Song period, the authorities had become very concerned by the incompetence of acupuncture specialists, who often applied acupuncture or moxibustion at the wrong location. In his preface to Wang Weiyi's manual, the official Xia Song 夏竦 (985–1051), for instance, denounced the errors made by practitioners in their clinical practice, which, he contended, resulted from the lack of reliability of the medical classics used as training manuals.[13] Wang Weiyi's textbook, whose compilation was ordered by the emperor Renzong 仁宗 (1010–1063), aimed at standardizing the number of circulation channels, their course on the body, and the number of acupuncture points belonging to each channel. This textbook was conceived both as a handbook for clinical practice and as a manual to accompany the bronze figures representing the acupuncture points.[14] This combination of Wang Weiyi's manual and the bronze figures was innovative, for the training of acupuncture specialists no longer had to rely only on a textual description of the channels and the acupuncture points but also used multimedia pedagogical tools.[15]

Under the supervision of the Bureau for Emending Medical Texts (Jiaozheng yishu ju 校正醫書局), established in 1057, several classical works compiled during the Han dynasty were revised and published in response to a new wave of epidemics. Three of them concerned acupuncture knowledge: the *Zhenjiu jiayi jing* 針灸甲乙經 (*The Classic of Acupuncture and Moxibustion in One, Two [Three ... Juan]*), the *Huangdi neijing suwen* 黃帝內經素問 (*The Yellow Emperor's Inner Classic: Basic Questions*), and the *Huangdi neijing*

---

11   Wang Tao 王燾 (670–755), the author of the *Waitai miyao fang* 外臺秘要方 (*Secret and Essential Formulas from the Royal Library*, 752) and a fervent advocate of moxibustion, strongly opposed acupuncture, for it could kill a man. See Yu 2007, 322.

12   In the preface of the Dunhuang moxibustion charts, the author explains, for instance, that he collected moxibustion prescriptions to provide a practical medicine for those living in remote regions and those who had no access to sophisticated drugs. See Lo 2005, 233. See also Yu 2007, 325–326.

13   Goldschmidt 2005, 66.

14   The content of Wang Weiyi's manual is described in Ma 1993, 91.

15   Bray, Dorofeeva-Lichtmann, and Métailié 2007, 29.

lingshu. There had been already several attempts in the past to revise these classics, such as Yang Shangshan's 楊上善 and Wang Bing's 王氷 annotated version of what was then thought to be the complete *Huangdi neijing*, but the previous revisions never achieved a position of authority and lost their importance after the fall of the Tang dynasty. On the other hand, the Bureau for Emending Medical Texts, an official organ directly sponsored by the imperial court, produced revised versions of these medical classics that became reference texts for all current extant editions.[16] Their dissemination benefited both from the development of printing technology and from the authorities' encouragement of the pursuit of a medical career for candidates who failed the civil service examination. It favored the emergence of a new group of literati physicians whose education and legitimacy were based on their expertise in the medical classics.[17] Following this revival of classical medicine, acupuncture regained its prominence in clinical practice, whereas moxibustion— which was a rather painful therapy since the moxa were burned directly on the skin—declined gradually.[18]

Interestingly, these changes in the medical field in China during the Song dynasty did not have any immediate influence on Japanese acupuncture until the late sixteenth century. Moxibustion never ceased to be popular during the Kamakura (1185–1333) and Muromachi (1337–1573) periods as a cheap and readily available therapy. During this period of turmoil and constant warfare waged by professional soldiers, moxa even became an essential item of warriors' equipment and was used on the battlefield to stop bleeding.[19] Its use by nonspecialists was so common that some authors warned against its abuse.[20] Although the channels theory is mentioned in Japanese medical textbooks written during these two periods and thus reflected some of the development of Chinese acupuncture during the Song dynasty, as in the Heian period there is little evidence that Japanese physicians applied it in their clinical practice. This suggests therefore that the transmission of the new Song knowledge on the channels theory was limited to a textual transmission of theoretical knowledge. Japanese physicians lacked the clinical training necessary to use acupuncture as a routine procedure.[21] This is particularly evident when comparing

---

16   Kosoto 2009, 212–219.

17   On the medical reforms during the Song dynasty, see Goldschmidt 2005, 69–73.

18   Yu 2007.

19   Fukunishi 2000, 41. Tominokōji's *Kikō* has a chapter dedicated to the treatment of battle-field wounds by moxibustion. See Goble 2011, 98.

20   Myōan (1211) 1994, 319–320.

21   The only illustration of a medieval physician administering a needle-based treatment appears in the *Yamai no sōshi* 病草紙 (Heian and Kamakura period). The illustration is

the chapters related to medical theory with those related to clinical practice in three of the most important medical textbooks compiled in medieval Japan: Kajiwara Shōzen's *Ton'ishō* 頓醫抄 (*Handbook for the Simple Physician*, 1304) and *Man'anpō* 萬安方 (*Formulas for Absolute Safety*, 1327) and Yūrin's *Fukuden hō* 福田方 (*Fukuden Formulary*, 1363).[22] Wang Weiyi's *Tongren yuxue zhenjiu tu jing*, first mentioned by Shōzen in his *Man'anpō* and whose role was central in China in the revival of classical acupuncture and the standardization of acupuncture points, did not have any influence on Japanese acupuncture other than providing a new source for textual study. Shōzen and Yūrin seem to have been unaware of its importance in China, and the fact that three other copies were transmitted to Japan before the seventeenth century was probably the result of the text's popularity in China rather than its popularity in Japan.[23]

Teaching What Classic? Manase Dōsan's Exegetical Study of Song and Ming Acupuncture Texts

In the historiography of Japanese medicine, Manase Dōsan is commonly regarded as having opened a new era for Japanese medicine by promulgating and disseminating via his school the theories of Li Dongyuan 李東垣 (1180/81–1251/52) and Zhu Danxi 朱丹溪 (1281–1358), two physicians of the Jin (1115–1234) and Yuan (1271–1368) periods whose works had been first introduced in

---

supposed to represent a physician applying acupuncture to a patient. However, this image is controversial, for it is not part of the original twenty illustrations of the *Yamai no sōshi* dating from the Heian period. It was added later (scholars agree that it is a work of the Kamakura period), along with an illustration representing a man suffering from hallucinations. Almost all features of the image (dimensions, format, technique, facial expressions) have no counterparts in the original drawings. In contrast to the original twenty illustrations, no text is provided, and it is difficult to determine from the image whether the needle is being inserted into the skin locally or at an acupuncture point, or even if it is being used for bloodletting or for pricking an abscess. Since other textual sources of the same period, such as the *Ton'ishō*, *Man'anpō*, and *Fukuden hō*, suggest that acupuncture (i.e., a needle applied to acupuncture points) was not used in clinical practice, it is most likely that this illustration represents a physician using a needle as a kind of surgical tool rather than for acupuncture. On the origin of this image, see Sano 1981, 1039: 7–28. On the relation between this illustration and the others, see Teramoto 1994.

22   Kajiwara Shōzen and Yūrin discussed the circulation channels theory separately from the acupuncture points and treatment. Their textbooks thus provide information on their exegetical, rather than their clinical, engagement with Chinese textual sources.

23   One copy was brought to Japan by Takeda Shōkei 竹田昌慶 (1338–1380) in 1363 along with replicas of the bronze figures, and the other two were transmitted in 1454 and 1533. On the dates of their transmission, see Mayanagi 2001.

Japan by Tashiro Sanki 田代三喜 (1465–1537).[24] Dōsan offered a radical departure from previous periods, for, in his work, acupuncture is not mentioned in passing in general compilations, as in Shōzen's and Yūrin's textbooks, but is an object of thorough study and teaching in its own right.[25] Dōsan spoke critically of the hyperspecialization of medicine that dominated both medical theory and practice and that ultimately created a culture in which physicians mastered only a single therapy. Acupuncture, moxibustion, and pharmacopeia formulas, Dōsan argued, were complementary therapies and should not be used independently from each other.[26] Dōsan was also concerned with the state of acupuncture in Japan, particularly the growing incompetence of acupuncture specialists:

> Suichiku Kusai's [i.e., Manase Dōsan] *Shinkyū shūyō* in one volume is a selection of the sages' *Shinkyū kei* [i.e., *Lingshu*] and *Jūyonkei* [i.e., *Shisijing fahui*]. Recently, acupuncture is employed arbitrarily. [Acupuncturists] do not know the course of the channels, the location of the acupuncture points, the acupuncture and moxibustion prohibitions, the gravity of diseases, the good and bad signs of the pulse, the taboos regarding application of acupuncture, [the consequences of] a wrong insertion; and no matter whether they are young or old, or whether they understand acupuncture theories or not, they all practice acupuncture. I think this is profoundly pathetic. Therefore, I have compiled [this textbook] in one volume. Those in this realm whose occupation is acupuncture must necessarily examine it.[27]

> 雖知苦齋針灸集要一卷者、是拔集諸聖賢是針灸經並十四經等者也。頃紊用針治而、不辨經升降所在、針灸禁、病淺深、脉吉凶、時月戒、刺巨繆而、少壯明晴俱懷針。予深憐焉。故撰彼一卷。天下業針之士、必須察之云。

His school in Kyoto, the Keiteki-in 啓迪院, was perhaps not only the first private school in Japan to train disciples on such a large scale but also the first,

---

24   On the Dōsan school, see Yakazu 1982; Endō 2007.

25   See, e.g., Nagano 2001a, 59–60. Machi (2008) analyzes the different editions of the *Shisijing fahui* circulating in Japan in the late sixteenth to early seventeenth centuries, including those consulted by Dōsan. See also Vigouroux 2011, 23–50.

26   Manase 1995, 353–354. Dōsan also insisted on the importance of an appropriate diet when the nutritive or defensive *qi* was deficient or when taking a treatment. See precepts 29 and 47 in his *Kirigami* (1979b, 7–14).

27   *Tōryū i no gen'i* 1777, 12. A similar passage is included in "Dōsan kafu" 1661.

since the Ishitsu-ryō 醫疾令 (Medical Laws) promulgated during the Nara period (710–794), to include a course on acupuncture.[28] Dōsan must have regarded acupuncture as a specialist knowledge, for in the nine-grade program of study in the Keiteki-in, acupuncture was taught only from the fifth grade on, after students had acquired some basic knowledge on diagnosis, remedies, and materia medica.[29]

Dōsan compiled several acupuncture manuals to be used as teaching resources—including manuals containing secret methods and aimed at a limited audience of disciples—but only three of the five textbooks he wrote are still extant: the *Shinkyū shūyō* 針灸集要 (*Essentials of Acupuncture and Moxibustion*, 1562), the *Shinkyū shinanshū* 針灸指南集 (*Instructions for Acupuncture and Moxibustion*), and the *Hikyū* 秘灸 (*Secret Moxibustion*). The two manuals no longer extant—the *Kinshinkyū ketsukai narabi gyōfuku dōshin sunhō* 禁針灸穴解並仰伏同身法 (*Prohibition of Acupuncture and Moxibustion Followed by a Supplement on the Measurement Method of the Body*, 1578), and the *Shinji seihō* 針治聖法 (*Divine Methods of Acupuncture Treatment*, 1582)—are only mentioned in the *Tōryū i no gen'i* 當流醫之源委 (*On the Origin of Our School*), a manuscript attributed to the Dōsan school, and in the *Dōsan kafu* 道三家譜 (*Genealogy of the Dōsan Family*).[30] Two short notes in the *Tōryū i no gen'i* explain that the *Kinshinkyū ketsukai narabi gyōfuku dōshin sunhō* was written in 1578 and the *Shinji seihō* was the result of a request from an acupuncturist named Shōkō Koji, who asked Dōsan to list in a single volume all the important acupuncture and moxibustion points.[31] Two textbooks listed in the nine-grades program bear similar titles; thus, it is likely that Dōsan used the *Kinshinkyū ketsukai narabi gyōfuku dōshin sunhō* and the *Shinji seihō* as teaching manuals in his school.[32]

The *Shinkyū shūyō* is the first Japanese textbook devoted solely to acupuncture and moxibustion, and it is also the only one of the three manuals still extant that provides detailed information about Dōsan's engagement with Song medical texts related to acupuncture. Divided into two parts, one explaining medical theories and the other more oriented toward clinical practice, the

---

28   Macé 1994a, 152.

29   *Tōryū i no gen'i* 1777, 7.

30   Although the manuscript is dated 1777, some passages were probably written by Dōsan himself. See Endō and Nakamura 1999, 337.

31   *Tōryū i no gen'i* 1777, 13.

32   In the sixth grade, students had to study the *Shinkyu kinketsu kai* 針灸禁穴解 (*Explanation of the Forbidden Acupuncture and Moxibustion Points*) and, in the seventh grade, the *Shinji seiden* 針治聖傳 (*The Sagely Tradition of Acupuncture Treatment*). See *Tōryū i no gen'i* 1777, 7.

Shinkyū shūyō contains 145 topics. All topics follow the same pattern: topic title, one character indicating the medical classic on which the topic is based, a
direct quotation (that sometimes includes a quotation of another classic), and
an explanatory diagram summarizing the topic. Thirteen medical classics are
cited—twelve Chinese and one Japanese—but most of the citations are drawn
from only five works: *Xushi zhenjiu daquan* 徐氏針灸大全 (*Mr. Xu's Comprehensive Collection of Acupuncture and Moxibustion*, 1439), *Zhenjiu ju ying* 針
灸聚英 (*Quintessence of Acupuncture and Moxibustion*, 1529), *Zhenjiu jieyao*
針灸節要 (*Essentials of Acupuncture and Moxibustion*, 1531), *Yilin leizheng
jiyao* 医林類証集要 (*Classified Compilation of the Medical Forest*, 1515), and
Zenkyūshū 全九集 (*Complete Nine Volumes*). Those five texts represent 85 percent of the 146 citations.

Although it was common practice in Chinese and Japanese writings to rely
on indirect citation when authors did not have physical access to the books—
this is particularly true for large compilations dealing with hundreds of citations—Dōsan cited from a relatively small number of classics that were
presumably readily accessible to him.[33] Cross-references in other documents
confirm that Dōsan consulted even the classics that he cited only once or
twice, and sometimes those he cited indirectly (i.e., in several topics Dōsan
quotes a passage that includes a quotation from another book).[34] Furthermore, all direct quotations are from textbooks written no earlier than the Song
dynasty, and in some cases, such as for the *Zhenjiu ju ying* or the *Zhenjiu jieyao*,
the classics are mentioned only a few years after their publication in China.

The *Shinkyū shūyo* is written as a vade mecum that practitioners could refer
to at all times. It is rather short, one volume written in the Chinese script with
reading marks, and Dōsan structured its contents in such a way that topics
could be read independently, but with the intention of covering all basic theoretical and practical knowledge necessary to the practice of acupuncture. Each
topic is written in a terse, concise manner, avoiding peripheral explanations,
and often Dōsan concludes with an explanatory diagram to sum up the citation.[35] In citing only texts from the Song and Ming dynasties, Dōsan clearly attempted to avoid superfluous repetition between classics, for Chinese

33   Goble 2011, 31.

34   The *Tōryū i no gen'i*, for instance, indicates that when Dōsan was fifteen years old, he
      studied the *Yu ji wei yi*, which he cites once in the *Shinkyū shūyō*. He also studied the
      Suwen, and in the entry on the administration of acupuncture in the *Shinkyū shūyō*,
      Dōsan cites a passage from the *Zhenjiu jieyao* that includes a quotation from the *Suwen*.
      See *Tōryū i no gen'i* 1777, 2.

35   The diagrams in the entries of the *Shinkyū shūyō* are similar to those in his *kirigami*. Com-
      pare, e.g., Manase 1995, 353–354, with Manase 1979b, 13, 22, 154.

classics from these two periods often cited earlier works. This editorial strategy enhanced the content of the text and gave the reader access to both the original text and the Song and Ming commentaries. Furthermore, Dōsan's emphasis on the latest Ming texts provided the reader with the most recent Chinese medical knowledge available in Japan.

Rubrics on the circulation channels theory and acupuncture convey a sense of the impact that Ming medical texts had on fifteenth-century Japanese medicine. Yet, in comparison with other documents related to the Dōsan school, the *Shinkyū shūyō* marks an early stage in Dōsan's appropriation of the circulation channels theory and acupuncture points. Most citations in these topics are drawn from the *Xushi zhenjiu daquan* and the *Zhenjiu ju ying*, although other sources are used to augment information, suggesting that at that stage Dōsan was still engaged in sorting out texts that could be used as teaching material in his school. This explains perhaps why he relied mostly on general compilations rather than on specialist textbooks. There is no reference, for instance, to Wang Weiyi's *Tongren yuxue zhenjiu tu jing*, although an obscure passage in the *Tōryū i no gen'i* indicates that Dōsan might have had access to it.[36] The *Shisijing fahui* is the only specialist text exclusively devoted to the circulation channels theory and the location of acupuncture points cited in the *Shinkyū shūyō*. Indeed, this is the first mention in Japan of this short manual written by the Chinese physician Hua Shou and first published in 1341 during the Yuan period.[37] However, the *Shisijing fahui* was not regarded yet as fundamental, for it is cited only twice in reference to minor subjects—the topics "Number of Points of the Channels" (諸經之穴数) and "Different Points, Same Name" (異穴同名).[38]

Two of Manase Dōsan's notes, *kirigami* 切紙 (lit. "paper strips"), compiled in 1571, nine years after the *Shinkyū shūyō*, provide additional information on what knowledge of the channels theory Dōsan taught to his disciples. The first note is divided into several paragraphs, each paragraph dealing with one particular topic: the six channels of the hand and foot, the fifteen collateral channels, the five command points of the twelve channels, the difference in the quantities of blood and *qi* in the twelve channels, the points of the back part of the body, the circulation of the conception channel, the four points for general treatments, prohibited points, and reunion points.[39] The content of these

---

36   *Tōryū i no gen'i* 1777, 6.

37   Two passages in the *Tōryū i no gen'i* refer also to Hua Shou's textbook. See *Tōryū i no gen'i* 1777, 3, 6.

38   Manase 1995, 409, 421.

39   Manase 1979b, 33–41.

paragraphs is similar to several rubrics of the *Shinkyū shūyō*, albeit expressed in a more concise form and with no reference to the Chinese classics. Most of these paragraphs, which are written in verse 歌, functioned as mnemonic aids to help students memorize the order of and specific instructions for the channels and points. Indeed, their content is not easily intelligible in itself, for no commentary is provided, and they make sense only when regarded as a textual aid to supplement the oral dimension of Dōsan's teaching. The verse "Song of the Four Chief Treatment Points" 四穴総治之歌 is an example of this "rhymed medical knowledge":[40]

> For the abdomen, halt at Sanli,
> For the lumbus and the back, search at Weizhong,
> For the head and the nape, inquire about Lieque,
> For the face and mouth, collect at Hegu.[41]

肚腹三里留
腰背委中求
頭項尋列缺
面口合谷收

The second *kirigami* is a diagram that spans two pages and is titled "Diagram of the Circulation of the Nutritive and Defensive [*qi*] Following or Against the Flow of the Twelve Channels" 十二經脉栄衛流注迎隨逆之圖. The six channels of the hand and the six channels of the feet are listed in three columns with their entry and exit points, linked together by a thin line to convey an image of the nutritive and defensive *qi* traveling from channel to channel and pervading the whole body. A short note on the circulation of the *qi* in the two main extraordinary channels based on the *Shisijing fahui* is appended with a final remark on the six Chinese medical texts on which Dōsan relied on to formulate his diagram. It suggests that nine years after the *Shinkyū shūyō*, Dōsan was still comparing Chinese sources, and no authoritative source on the circulation channels theory stood out from the others.[42] Yet, in 1574, three years

---

40 This tradition of writing in verse goes back to the Han dynasty (206 BCE–220 CE). As Rosalind Thomas (cited in Brashier 2005, 259) points out about the role of verse in ancient Greece: "anything passed on in verse has a better chance of accurate transmission." I also borrow the expression "rhymed medical knowledge" from Brashier 2005.

41 Manase 1979b, 37.

42 Dōsan (Manase 1979b, 104) explains that he created this diagram based on his understanding of the *Shisijing fahui, Xushi zhenjiu daquan, Ming tang jiu jing, Zhenjiu ju ying, Zhenjiu jieyao,* and the *Taiping shenghui fang.*

after these two *kirigami* were composed, Dōsan wrote a postscript to a short manuscript titled *Kōtei meidō kyū kei fushin shōshō* 黄帝明堂灸經不審少々 (*Some Doubts on the Moxibustion Classic of the Numinous Hall of the Yellow Emperor*) stating: "The explanations of the [Elucidation of the] Fourteen [Channels] classic are the only reference [to the channels theory]" 十四經之説、為定矩而已.[43] Nagano Hitoshi argues that this turning point in Dōsan's process of inquiry was his encounter with Hata Sōha 秦宗巴 (1549–1610), who entered his school around 1572.[44]

Information on Hata Sōha's life is fragmentary.[45] According to Asada Sōhaku 浅田宗伯 (1815–1894), who included a biography in the *Kōku mei'i den* 皇國名醫傳 (*Legends of Famous Doctors from Our Imperial Country*, 1851), Hata Sōha completed his medical training with Dōsan after having been recommended by his first master, Yoshida Sōkei 吉田宗桂 (?–1572), and later served as physician to Toyotomi Hidetsugu 豊臣秀次 (1568–1595).[46] Although he is perhaps best known for writing the *Tsurezuregusa Junyōin shō* 徒然草壽命院抄 (*Commentary of Junyōin on the Essays in Idleness*, 1604), the first commentary on the fourteenth-century *Tsurezuregusa*, Hata Sōha is also the author of two other important medical texts: a commentary on Ma Shi's 馬蒔 *Suwen zhu zheng fa wei* 素問注證發微 (*The Suwen, Commentated, Validated, and Elucidated*, 1586; Hata Sōha was the first person in Japan to lecture on Ma Shi's annotated edition of the *Suwen*) and the *Yuketsu sango teki hō* 俞穴参伍的法 (*Method for Classifying the Acupuncture Points*).[47]

The *Yuketsu sango teki hō* contains a postscript written by Dōsan and dated 1574, the same year as the postscript to the *Kōtei meidō kyū kei fushin shōshō*. Dōsan presents Hata Sōha's textbook as a synthesis of his exegetical study of Chinese medical texts, arguing that his manual is a "treasure that can bring back to life the dead."[48] Since the *Yuketsu sango teki hō* is a manuscript on acupuncture points whose content is based on Hua Shou's *Shisijing fahui*, Hata Sōha's arrival at the Keiteki-in must have been a factor in triggering Dōsan's research on the channels and acupuncture points; two years earlier, in 1572, when Dōsan wrote his *kirigami* on circulation channels theory, the *Shisijing*

43   *Kōtei meidō kyū kei fushin shōshō* (1574), n.p.

44   Nagano 2001a, 60.

45   Hata Sōha seems to have been well acquainted with some of the aristocratic families of the Kyoto court, as he appears in many entries of the *Tokitsune kyōki* 言経卿記 (Tokitsune's diary), the journal of the aristocrat-physician Yamashina Tokitsune 山科言経 (1543–1611). However, Yamashina (1959–1991, 5:35) records in his journal that he first met Hata on March 20, 1592. On Yamashina, see also Goble 2008.

46   Asada (1851) 1983, 347–350.

47   On the *Tsurezuregusa Junyōin shō*, see Keene 1976, 138.

48   Nagano 2001a, 60.

fahui was still listed as one source among others. The *Kōtei meidō kyū kei fushin shōshō* must be regarded therefore as Dōsan's and Hata Sōha's reevaluation of Chinese medical texts and the *Yuketsu sango teki hō* as the result of their inquiry. That is, Hua Shou's *Shisijing fahui* was selected as the only reliable text for transmitting the channels theory and the location of acupuncture points.

Dōsan's knowledge of acupuncture was certainly more advanced than that of his medieval predecessors. Yet his acupuncture manuals and *kirigami* indicate only what theoretical knowledge he gained from Song and Ming medical texts. The question remains of whether he incorporated this knowledge into his clinical practice, or whether his clinical practice helped him to identify shortcomings in these texts. In others words, how did Dōsan correlate theoretical knowledge learned from texts with knowledge learned from clinical encounters with patients? This question is difficult to answer because Dōsan did not keep any detailed clinical records dealing with acupuncture therapy.[49] Although he might have relied on his personal clinical experience to validate the theoretical knowledge he gained from the medical classics mentioned in the *Shinkyū shūyō*, this textbook is an attempt to adapt existing knowledge to a different context, not a groundbreaking work producing new knowledge. Its originality lies more in the arrangement of the different subjects (number, topic, citation) than on their content. Even the second part, which deals with acupuncture treatments, does not offer much opportunity for learning about Dōsan's clinical experience, for, like the first part, the entries merely consist of citations. There is no description of the disease (symptoms, characteristics of the pulse, evolution), only the treatment. The entry on dizziness 頭眩 is an instructive example:

> Dizziness [*Shanghan*] *zhili*
> Apply acupuncture to [the points] Shangxing [*j.* Jōsei, GV23], Fengchi [*j.* Fūchi, GB20], and Tianzhu [*j.* Tenchū, BL10].
> The *Shouyu shenfang* says: apply moxibustion [to the points] Tianzhu [*j.* Tenchū, BL10] and Tongtian [*j.* Tsūten, BL10]. [Insert] needles 3 *fen* and [apply] three cones of moxa.[50]

> 頭眩 治例
> 針上星風池天柱
> 寿域曰灸天枢通天針三分灸三壮

---

49 His *Shusshō haizai* 出証配剤 (*Formulas Given according to Symptoms*) is the only record of case histories left by Dōsan, but it deals mostly with formula treatments, although he also mentions application of moxa to specific points for a few cases. See Manase 1979c.

50 Manase 1995, 440.

In this example, the main part is a citation from the *Shanghan zhili* (*Case Treatments of Cold Damage Disorders*), which is augmented by an optional treatment from the *Shouyu shenfang*. Therefore, the type of afflictions mentioned is perhaps the only evidence of Dōsan's clinical experience, for it is most likely that Dōsan recorded the most common afflictions he encountered in his clinical practice. In any case, the content of the rubric suggests that the reader already has the basic knowledge to diagnose dizziness, since only information on the treatment is provided. This explains perhaps why acupuncture began to be taught only once the student had reached the fifth grade in Dōsan's school—that is, as specialist knowledge learned after the core program covering basic medical knowledge on disease and diagnosis had been mastered.

Overall, in Dōsan's works there is no sharp difference from previous periods regarding the frequency of moxibustion and acupuncture treatment. Moxibustion is still mentioned more often than acupuncture. Out of a total of fifty-four diseases, moxibustion is recommended forty-nine times, acupuncture sixteen times, and bloodletting two times in the second part of the *Shinkyū shūyō*. Only in three cases is acupuncture the single treatment. In thirteen cases, acupuncture is always administered in combination with moxibustion. Bloodletting is mentioned the first time in combination with moxibustion, and the second time in combination with acupuncture and moxibustion. A comparison with Dōsan's most famous compendium on diagnosis and therapy confirms the domination of moxibustion treatment over acupuncture. In the *Keiteki shū* 啓迪集 (*Compendium of the Keiteki*), acupuncture and moxibustion are mentioned as complementary therapies to herbal remedies in the treatment of sixteen afflictions: in two cases only acupuncture is employed, in nine cases only moxibustion, and in five cases they are administered together. However, acupuncture therapy is administered on specific acupuncture points only for the treatment of three afflictions. In one case, acupuncture is recommended in combination with moxibustion but without information on how to administer it. In the last three cases, needles are applied locally either for bloodletting, opening abscesses using the fire needle technique, or stopping verbal delirium by puncturing the nail bed.[51]

This domination of moxibustion therapy was not particular to Dōsan; other sources from the same period provide a similar picture.[52] Moreover, since

---

51   Manase (1571) 1979a, 2:73–77, 312–313, 351, 363, 368, 407–408, 419–420, 432, 445, 532–533; 3:36, 49, 57, 80, 155–156, 178–179, 351–358.

52   See, for example, the *Tamon-in nikki* 多聞院日記 (*Journal of Tamon-in*), the journal of the monk Eishun 英俊 (1518–1596) of the temple Kōfukuji 興福寺. Many entries record that Eishun frequently resorted to moxibustion therapy to relieve chronic eye infections

both the *Shinkyū shūyō* and the *Keiteki-shū* are compilations of Song and Ming medical texts, their emphasis on moxibustion reflects Chinese medical practice as much as it does sixteenth-century Japanese medical practice, suggesting that the revival of classical acupuncture and the shift from moxibustion to acupuncture during the Song dynasty was probably less radical than has been argued by some scholars.[53] Furthermore, since the *Shinkyū shūyō* and the *Keiteki shū* were both compiled before Hata Sōha's arrival at the Keiteki-in, it is not possible to know how much Dōsan's reevaluation of the Song and Ming medical texts in the 1570s, and as a result his adoption of the *Shisijing fahui* as the reference text for teaching the circulation channels theory and acupuncture points, influenced his clinical practice toward the end of his life.

Concurrently with Dōsan's scholarly interest in sorting out acupuncture theories to compile reliable teaching materials for his students, the sixteenth century witnessed the emergence of new acupuncture schools that developed new theories outside the framework of the circulation channels theory. In the late sixteenth century, Mubun 夢分, for instance, invented a new technique of insertion called the hammer technique (*uchi-bari* 打針), which involved inserting needles into the skin with a small wooden hammer. He passed on this technique to Misono Isai 御薗意斎 (1557–1616), the founder of the Misono school, and it came to be used only on the abdomen area, the receptacle of the five viscera and the six bowels, regarded as the seat of all diseases.[54] Information on the origin of the *uchi-bari* technique is scarce, but it seems likely to be an adaptation of a fifteenth-century horticultural technique originally used to kill insects and worms in trees by puncturing them with a punch.[55] Interestingly, the appearance of this technique coincided with a new notion that afflictions were caused by insects and worms. The *Hari kikigaki* 針聞書 (*An Account of Things Heard about Acupuncture*), written in 1568 by Ibaragi Gengyō 茨木元行, the founder of the Konshin school 今新, includes sixty-three illustrations

---

and buboes; only a few mention acupuncture. See Eishun 1978, 2:203, 457; 3:424; 4:179; 5:13. See also Vigouroux 2011, 46–47.

53   See, e.g., Yu 2007. Asaf Goldschmidt (2009, 30–41) contends that the publication of Wang Weiyi's textbook had a great impact on the revival of classical medicine, but he regards acupuncture and moxibustion as a single therapy—acu-moxa—without explaining how the clinical use of acupuncture and moxibustion as distinct therapies evolved from previous periods.

54   On the Misono school, see *Misono ie rekiden ryakki* 1989. On their mapping of the abdomen area, see *Shindō hiketsu shū* 1978, 3–4.

55   Shōsei Saidōtan 樵青洞丹 (1994, 10) mentions in his *Enrashi shinkyū hō* 煙蘿子針灸法 (*Enrashi's Acupuncture and Moxibustion Methods*), written in 1530, the story of a horticulturist using a punch to kill the insects that were attacking trees.

of parasites divided into six categories according to their forms.[56] However, not all the new acupuncture schools focused on the abdomen area. A recently discovered manuscript of the Irie school 入江, whose founder Irie Yoriaki 入江 頼明 served Toyotomi Hideyoshi 豊臣秀吉 (1536–1537) during his Korean campaign in 1592 and remained for four years in Chosŏn Korea to study acupuncture under the Ming physician Gō Rintatsu 呉林達, contained several drawings of the human body describing the acupuncture points without any reference to the channels.[57]

Appropriation and Innovation: The *Shisijing Fahui* and Tokugawa Acupuncture

Only two editions of the *Shisijing fahui* circulated in Japan during the Tokugawa period. One was the revised version of the 1369 edition by the Imperial College physician Xue Kai 薛鎧 published in 1528 by his son Xue Ji 薛己 (1487–1559) in his *Xue shi yi an* 薛氏醫案 (*Mr. Xue's Medical Case Records*). This edition was most likely the edition that Manase Dōsan and Hata Sōha mentioned in their writings, although we do not know how they gained access to it. The second edition was a Korean edition transmitted during Toyotomi Hideyoshi's campaigns in Korea in 1592 and 1598.

Printing technology played an important role in the diffusion in Japan of the *Shisijing fahui* after Dōsan proclaimed its superiority over other textbooks for learning the circulation channels theory. Indeed, it is not a coincidence that the first Japanese edition of the *Shisijing fahui* was printed in movable type 古活字 in 1598 by the literati physician Oze Hoan 小瀬甫庵 (1564–1640), a member of the inner circle of the Manase family. This edition has been lost. The earliest Japanese edition extant is a 1604 reprint of the Korean edition.[58] In total, Hua Shou's textbook was reprinted twenty-one times during the Tokugawa period (1604, 1618, 1625, 1631, 1649, 1660, 1665, 1675, 1684, 1695, 1709, 1716, 1731, 1762, 1764, 1796, 1798, 1801, 1805, 1806, 1839). It is difficult, however, to assess the significance of the number of times that Hua Shou's textbook was imported, because that number corresponds to the number of times that the *Xue shi yi an* was imported (twelve times: 1638, 1710, 1719, 1722, 1725, 1735, 1759, 1837, 1839, 1844, 1845, 1849). This number most likely indicates the popularity of Xue Ji's

---

56   On this book, see *Mushi no shirase* 2007; Nagano and Higashi 2007.

57   *Kaiden Irieryū shinjutsu* 2002.

58   Senjurō Machi (2008, 47) argues that the publisher also consulted the Chinese version to make corrections.

book among Japanese physicians due to its coverage of all domains of Chinese medicine rather than specifically Xue's inclusion of the revised version of Hua Shou's textbook. The numerous Japanese reprints of either the Chinese or the Korean edition show an expanding domestic demand for the original text, but also suggest that as a result the text circulated widely in Japan, and therefore, it was not necessary to import the Chinese or Korean editions, particularly because no new editions were printed in China or Korea. By comparison, Wang Weiyi's *Tongren yuxue zhenjiu tu jing* was only imported once (1694) and published once (1654) during the Tokugawa period based on an earlier edition.[59]

Tamura Gensen's 谷村玄仙 *Jushikei hakki shō* 十四經發揮抄 (*Elucidation of the Fourteen Channels Annotated*), published in 1661, was the first Japanese commentary on Hua Shou's *Shisijing fahui*—and was one of the longest commentaries written during the Tokugawa period: 389 leaves in ten volumes, whereas the original edition was only 69 leaves in one volume. Thus, it took sixty years after the *Shisijing fahui* was printed for the first time in Japan before a Japanese physician produced a commentary edition—one hundred years if we include its first mention in Dōsan's *Shinkyū shūyō*. Stressing the importance of the channels theory, Tamura compares the physician who does not know the channels theory to "a person walking during the night without a candle."[60] The publication of Tamura's *Jushikei hakki shō* spurred the production of commentated and annotated editions of Hua Shou's book, which were published either with reading marks (*kaeri ten* 返り点) or with readings of the Chinese characters (*okuri gana* 送り仮名) or were completely rewritten in vernacular Japanese, which significantly helped Japanese acupuncture practitioners to assimilate the rather complex channels theory during the seventeenth century.

Eight of these commentaries were published during the second half of the seventeenth century, indicating that Japanese physicians first learned the circulation channels theory from the original content before producing commentaries. Interestingly, all Chinese medical texts transmitted to Japan during the Tokugawa period did not follow the same process of dissemination. For instance, the figures regarding the importation and Japanese reprinting of textbooks related to the *Huangdi neijing* and the *Nanjing* 難經 (*Classic of Difficulties*) suggest that, unlike the case with the *Shisijing fahui*, Japanese physicians relied first on commentated editions before turning to the original text.[61]

---

59   On these imports and Japanese editions, see Vigouroux 2011, 98–130.

60   Quoted from Gabor (2010, 91), who presents in his book on marginalia in Japanese medical textbooks an edition of Tamura Gensen's *Jushikei hakki shō* that was annotated by hand.

61   Vigouroux 2011, 98–123.

Acupuncture mannequins and charts also became necessary components of the appropriation and dissemination of the circulation channels theory. The Song period physician Wang Weiyi was the first to acknowledge the importance of three-dimensional visual aids to complement textual sources for teaching acupuncture. In 1027 he commissioned the casting of two bronze figures on which the locations of acupuncture points were indicated. The figures were entirely covered with wax and filled with water; when the student accurately inserted the needle at the location of an acupuncture point, water poured out from the point.[62] Although a replica was brought to Japan as early as the fourteenth century, it did not have any impact in Japan until Japanese acupuncturists began to apply the channels theory to clinical practice in the early Tokugawa period. Indeed, the production of Japanese mannequins was concurrent with the publication of annotated and commentary editions of Hua Shou's *Shisijing fahui* in the second half of the seventeenth century.

Two major differences distinguished Japanese acupuncture mannequins from their Chinese counterparts: they were usually smaller and made of paper or wood.[63] These particular characteristics of the Japanese mannequins not only allowed Japanese physicians to represent the bones more accurately, particularly those of the thorax, and the course of the channels on the body but also made their production easier, and thus, acupuncture mannequins became relatively available. The Dutch physician Willem ten Rhyne (1647–1700), who lived in Japan for two years in the late 1670s, mentioned the popularity of these small acupuncture mannequins in his account on Japanese medicine, explaining that most acupuncturists had one on display outside their home to advertise their practice.[64] In 1690 the artisan category "acupuncture mannequin maker" (*dōjingyō shi* 銅人形師) even made its way into the *Jinrin kinmō zui* 人倫訓蒙図彙 (*Illustrated Encyclopedia of Humanity*), which gives the address of two such artisans in the cities of Osaka and Edo.[65]

---

62   Goldschmidt 2005, 67.

63   The two exceptions are the two bronze acupuncture figures held by the Tokyo National Museum and measuring, respectively, 143.9 and 161 centimeters. The first figure was made by Iimura Gensai 飯村玄斎 in 1662, and the second by Yamazaki Tsugiyoshi 山崎次善 when he was teaching at the *bakufu* Medical School (Igakkan 医学館) between 1789 and 1800. See Nagano 2001b; Kosoto 1989. Most of the wood and paper acupuncture figures included in Nagano 2001a measure less than 100 centimeters. The wood figure on display in the specimen room of Tokyo University Medical School is 87 centimeters. See Yōhō 1995, 44.

64   Rhyne 1683, 180.

65   *Jinrin kinmō zui* 1990, 190.

The Japanese acupuncture mannequins and charts were not mere copies of Chinese representations of the channels and acupuncture points. Japanese physicians visually innovated by depicting the reunion points, particularly those located on the abdomen area, to show the internal connections between channels and sometimes between channels and organs.[66] These depictions aimed at recording what was invisible to the eyes and yet essential to the clinical application of the circulation channels theory. This innovation also represented an attempt to merge the two different traditions that appeared in sixteenth-century Japanese acupuncture: one represented by the Dōsan school and focusing on the classic channels theory and one represented by the Misono school and focusing exclusively on the abdomen outside the framework of the channels and acupuncture points.

The visual accumulation of detail on the connections between channels and the functions of the points in the abdomen area made the charts and the mannequins illegible to untrained eyes. The mannequins and charts had to be decoded in conjunction with textual explanations to become functional.[67] As Brian Baigrie points out: "every diagram is a kind of encoding that demands a set of conventions that are shared by the illustrations and the user. If the user is unfamiliar with the conventions at work, this compromises their utility."[68] Therefore, these acupuncture charts and mannequins were not produced for popular pedagogy but were intended to communicate technical knowledge to already-practicing acupuncturists or to those training to become practitioners. To anyone trained to read them, these tools could serve as mnemonic devices that economically and instantaneously conveyed the complex trajectory and interconnections of the channels running on and below the surface of the body.

Reconsidering the Circulation Channels Theory in the Late Tokugawa Period

The vicissitudes of Chinese medical texts through the Tokugawa period mirrored intellectual trends in Chinese scholarship. The introduction of Qing evidential research methods particularly gave rise to a new "era of Japanese

---

66   Nagano (2001a) shows several of these Japanese acupuncture figures and charts made during the seventeenth and eighteenth centuries.

67   On the function of *tu* 圖 and the relation between text and image in China, see Bray, Dorofeeva-Lichtmann, and Métailié 2007.

68   Baigrie 1996, 11.

medical philology," offering Japanese physicians methodological and epistemological tools to reconsider Chinese medical knowledge directly from the
original texts without depending on later commentaries.[69] For example, the
physician Murai Kinzan 村井琴山 (1733–1815) made a philological study of
the first part of the *Huangdi neijing* based on a comparison of rhymes 韻語.
Phonological tools enabled him to argue that the original content of this work
had been distorted by the Tang physician Wang Bing and to conclude his analysis with what he thought were the original sixty-one chapters (instead of the
eighty-one chapters of Wang Bing's version), as indicated by Quan Yuanqi's 全
元起 *Suwen xun jie* 素問訓解 (*Basic Questions Commentary*)—the first known
commentated edition of the *Huangdi neijing*, which was compiled during the
sixth century.[70] This return to antiquity led eventually to the discrediting of the
Danxi synthesis[71] and the resurrection of the author of the *Shanghan lun* 傷寒
論 (*Treatise on Cold Damage Disorders*), the second-century physician Zhang
Zhongjing 張仲景, as the ultimate medical authority.

Influenced by this turn toward ancient medicine, during the eighteenth
century certain acupuncture practitioners started to express skepticism about
the efficacy of the channels theory without necessarily advocating the Misono
school approach, which focused on the abdomen area as the seat of all diseases. Suganuma Shukei 菅沼周桂, for instance, who was inspired by the work
of Yoshimasu Tōdō 吉益東洞 (1702–1773), one of the leading figures of the Ancient Formulas School (Kohō-ha 古方派), refuted the entire channels theory
and the theories about the forbidden points, the *yu* 俞 points, and the reunion
points, setting the number of regular acupuncture points to only seventy and
referring uniquely to anatomical marks to locate the points on the body.[72]

Other practitioners virulently attacked the eminence reached by Hua Shou's
textbook during the seventeenth century. As Hirose Hakurin 広瀬白鱗
claimed in his *Hi juyonkei ben* 非十四經辨 (*Arguments against the Fourteen
Channels*, 1775), they believed that Hua Shou had betrayed the teachings of the
ancient sages. Hua Shou's first unforgivable mistake was to have assimilated
the *dumai* 督脈 and *renmai* 任脈 channels to the twelve regular channels,
which in Hirose's eyes was the height of stupidity (愚昧ノ至也), for these two
channels are originally two of the eight extraordinary channels. Second, Hua
Shou advocated the method of localizing acupuncture points according to

---

69   Elman 2008, 110.

70   Murai Kinzan, *Idō nisennen ganmoku hen*, vol. 4. On Quan Yuanqi, see also Unschuld 2003,
      24–25.

71   See the essay by Fabien Simonis in this volume.

72   Suganuma (1767) 1978, 2.

anatomical benchmarks (骨度法) instead of using the ancient method of identical units of the body (同身寸法). The transmission of this "smelly rubbish" 糟粕餘臭 to later generations was responsible, Hirose contended, for the corruption of the acupuncture tradition in Japan.[73]

In the midst of the new thriving intellectual environment centered on Dutch medicine at the turn of the nineteenth century, the imperial acupuncturist Ishizaka Sōtetsu 石坂宗哲 (1770–1841) used the new cutting-edge knowledge of anatomy to rethink the circulation channels theory, assimilating the acupuncture channels to the Western blood and nerve systems.[74] The basic principle of acupuncture, he explained, is the inflammatory reaction following the insertion into the human body of a foreign object. The needle inserted into the affected part provoked a local inflammation, which stimulated the living *qi* and the blood under the needle to form the original *qi*, which then expelled the pathogenic agent from the body.[75] Neither the insertion of the acupuncture needle directly into the affected area nor the idea of expelling the evil agent from the body was new. What was innovative, however, was that Ishizaka Sōtetsu made application of acupuncture in *loco dolenti* a general principle of the circulation channels theory, and that his explanation of the action of the acupuncture needle did not present any significant problems of understanding to a mind educated in Western medicine. This explains why the German physician Philipp Franz von Siebold (1796–1866), who resided in Japan in the 1820s, had so much interest in Ishizaka Sōtetsu's theories.[76]

His medical ideas, however, did not represent a radical break with past Japanese acupuncture ideas. They took their place among the latest developments of the seventeenth- and eighteenth-century academic disputes that highlighted the symbolic struggles of Japanese physicians to reinterpret the textual tradition of Chinese medicine. Ishizaka Sōtetsu surely saw himself as the "true classicist" of the Tokugawa period, but he did so in the vein of many Japanese physicians long before him.[77] There is no evidence that he ever assisted in performing dissections, and his interpretations of Western anatomy treatises were very loose, adopting only concepts that fit his theories. These attitudes explain why he never considered Dutch medicine to be superior to the Chinese medi-

---

73 Hirose (1775) 1990, 6–9.
74 Macé (1994b) provides a full explanation of the charts held by the Bibliothèque nationale de France that represent Ishizaka Sōtetsu's attempt to assimilate the nutritive and defensive *qi* channels to the arteries and veins of Western medicine.
75 Ishizaka, ca. 1820–1825, n.p.
76 On Ishizaka and Siebold, see Kure 1931.
77 Elman 2008, 117.

cal tradition and even publicly condemned his peers who paid too much attention to the medicine of the "barbarians."[78]

Conclusion

The developments that acupuncture underwent in Japan during the Tokugawa period stand in stark contrast to its decline in Qing China. After the last Ming dynasty publications on acupuncture—*Shen ying jing* 神應經 (*Classic for Wondrous Response*) in 1425, *Zhenjiu ju ying* in 1529, and *Zhenjiu dacheng* 針灸大成 (*Great Compendium of Acupuncture and Moxibustion*) in 1601—acupuncture in China lost its prominent status among elite physicians and became a low-class therapy. It reached its lowest ebb in 1822, when the imperial authority decided to close the department of acupuncture at the Imperial College.[79]

The persistence of local traditions and the absence of an official organ responsible for standardizing medical knowledge and establishing authoritative texts, such as the Bureau for Emending Medical Texts in Song China, account for why Hua Shou's *Shisijing fahui* never achieved a prominent position in Japan and why Japanese acupuncturists continuously tried to adapt the circulation channels theory to their own theoretical framework.

Ironically, the Chinese only rediscovered Hua Shou's manual during the twentieth century thanks to the popularity it reached in Japan. During a visit to Tokyo in the 1930s, the Chinese physician Cheng Dan'an 承淡安 (1899–1957) noticed that the *Shisijing fahui* was used as a textbook in Japanese acupuncture schools. He decided to buy a Japanese edition, which he subsequently used to publish, in 1936, the first modern Chinese edition of this text.[80] This reprint of the *Shisijing fahui* and Makoto Mayanagi's essay in this volume on Yang Shoujing 楊守敬 (1839–1915), who also reprinted in China rare medical books that he had collected from the Kojima 小島 family during his stay in Japan in the 1880s, are two instructive examples illustrating the rather complex circulation of Chinese medical texts in East Asia.

---

78   Ishizaka (ca. 1815–1825) 1990, 446.

79   Peking chūigakuin hen 1964, 169; Lu and Needham 2002, 60.

80   His edition of the *Shisijing fahui* was a reprint of Tatsui Fumikata's 辰井文隆 1929 edition of Hatta Taikyō's 八田泰興 edition of the *Shisijing fahui*, first published in 1829. See Mayanagi 2006.

References

Asada Sōhaku 浅田宗伯 (1851) 1983. *Kōku mei'i den* 皇國名醫傳 [Legends of famous doctors from our imperial country], *Kinsei kanpō igakusho shūsei* 近世漢方医学書集成 99. Tokyo: Meicho shuppan.

Baigrie, Brian, ed. 1996. *Picturing Knowledge: Historical and Philosophical Problems concerning the Use of Art in Science*. Toronto: University of Toronto Press.

Barnes, Linda 2005. *Needles, Herbs, Gods, and Ghosts: China Healing and the West to 1848*. Cambridge, MA: Harvard University Press.

Brashier, Ken 2005. "Text and Ritual in Early Chinese Stelae," in Martin Kern, ed., *Text and Ritual in Early China*. Seattle: University of Washington Press, 249–283.

Bray, Francesca, Vera Dorofeeva-Lichtmann, and Georges Métailié, eds. 2007. *Graphics and Text in the Production of Technical Knowledge in China*. Leiden: E. J. Brill.

Cook, Harold 2007. *Matters of Exchange: Commerce, Medicine, and Science in the Dutch Golden Age*. New Haven, CT: Yale University Press.

——— 2011. "Conveying Chinese Medicine to Seventeenth-Century Europe," *Science between Europe and Asia* 275, 4: 209–232.

"Dōsan kafu" 道三家譜 [Genealogy of the Dōsan family] 1661. In Kaya Matsuan 加屋松庵, *Shōni ryōji shū* 小児療治集 [Compilation of treatments for children]. Kyoto: Tokuda Hatsuuemon. National Archives of Japan 国立公文館 (195–0243).

Eishun 英俊 (1534–1596) 1978. *Tamon-in nikki* 多聞院日記 [Journal of Tamon-in], in Takeuchi Rizō 竹内理三, ed., *Zoku shiryō taisei* 続史料大成 [Second series of historical materials]. Kyoto: Rinsen shoten.

Elman, Benjamin 2008. "Sinophiles and Sinophobes in Tokugawa Japan: Politics, Classicism, and Medicine during the Eighteenth Century," *East Asian Science, Technology, and Society: An International Journal* 2: 93–121.

Endō, Jirō 遠藤次郎 2007. "Manase Dōsan no igaku" 曲直瀬道三の医学 [The medicine of Manase Dōsan], *Kyōu* 杏雨 10: 125–140.

Endō Jirō 遠藤次郎 and Nakamura Teruko 中村輝子 1999. "Manase dōsan no zenhanki no igaku: Tōryū no igi" 曲直瀬道三の前半期の医学－「当流」の意義 [The medicine of the first period of Manase Dōsan: The meaning of "our school"], *Nihon ishigaku zasshi* 日本医史学雑誌 45, 3: 323–338.

Fukunishi Sukeharu 福西佐元 2000. *Okyū banashi arekore* お灸ばなしあれこれ [Various stories about moxibustion]. Tokyo: Iwanami shoten.

Gabor, Lukacs 2010. *Extensive Marginalia in Old Japanese Medical Books*. Piribebuy, Paraguay: Wayenborgh.

Goble, Andrew 2008. "Rhythms of Medicine and Community in Late Sixteenth Century Japan: Yamashina Tokitsune (1543–1611) and His Patients," *East Asian Science, Technology, and Medicine* 29: 13–61.

———— 2011. *Confluences of Medicine in Medieval Japan: Buddhist Healing, Chinese Knowledge, Islamic Formulas, and Wounds of War*. Honolulu: University of Hawai'i Press.

Goldschmidt, Asaf 2005. "Song Discontinuity: Rapid Innovation in Northern Song Dynasty Medicine," *Asian Medicine* 1, 1: 53–90.

———— 2009. *The Evolution of Chinese Medicine*. London: Routledge Curzon.

Harper, Donald 1998. *Early Chinese Medical Literature*. London: Kegan Paul International.

Hirose, Hakurin 広瀬白鱗 (1775) 1990. *Hijuyonkei ben* 非十四經辨 [Arguments against the fourteen channels], *Rinshō shinkyū koten zensho* 臨床鍼灸古典全書 21. Osaka: Oriento shuppansha.

Ishizaka Sōtetsu 石坂宗哲 (ca. 1815–1825) 1990. *Igen* 醫源 [On the origin of medicine], *Rinshō shinkyū koten zensho* 臨床鍼灸古典全書 16. Osaka: Oriental shuppansha.

———— ca. 1820–1825. *Chiyō ichigen* 知要一言 [Essentials of acupuncture in a few words]. Leiden University Library (UB1092).

Jinrin kinmō zui 人倫訓蒙図彙 [Illustrated encyclopedia of humanity] (1690) 1990. Tokyo: Heibonsha.

Kaiden Irieryū shinjutsu: Irie nakatsukasa sunaisuke onsōdenhari no sho no fukkoku to kenkyū 皆伝・入江流鍼術: 入江中務少輔御相伝針之書の覆刻と研究 [Initiation to the acupuncture of the Irie school: Research and reedition of the junior assistant of the Central Affairs Bureau Irie's book on the tradition of acupuncture] 2002. Edited by Ōura Jikan 大浦慈観 and Nagano Hitoshi 長野仁. Tokyo: Rokuzensha.

Kajiwara Shōzen's *Ton'ishō* 頓醫抄 (Handbook for the Simple Physician, 1304).

Keene, Donald 1976. *World within Walls: Japanese Literature of the Pre-modern Era, 1600–1867*. New York: Holt, Rinehart and Winston.

Kosoto Hiroshi 小曽戸洋 1989. "Tōhaku dōjinkei no seisakusha oyobi nendai ni tsuite" 東博銅人形の制作者および年代について [About the maker and the date of the bronze figure in the Tokyo National Museum], *Nihon ishigaku zasshi* 日本医史学雑誌 35, 2: 140–142.

———— 2009. "Volumes of Knowledge: Observations on Song-Period Printed Medical Texts," in Andrew E. Goble, Kenneth R. Robinson, and Haruko Wakabayashi, eds., *Tools of Culture: Japan's Cultural, Intellectual, Medical, and Technological Contacts in East Asia, 1000–1500s*. Ann Arbor: Association for Asian Studies, 212–219.

Kosoto Hiroshi 小曽戸洋, Seki Nobuyuki 関信之, and Kurihara Mariko 栗原萬里子 1990. "Wakokubon kanseki isho shuppan sōgō nenpyō" 和刻本漢籍医書出版総合年表 [Comprehensive chronology of Japanese edition of Chinese medicine books], *Nihon ishigaku zasshi* 日本医史学雑誌 36, 1: 459–494.

Kōtei meidō kyū kei fushin shōshō 黄帝明堂灸經不審少々 [Some doubts about the moxibustion classic of the Numinous Hall of the Yellow Emperor] 1574. Takeda kagaku shinkō zaidan kyōu shooku 武田科学振興財団杏雨書屋 (杏 5185).

Kure, Shūzō 呉秀三 1931. "Tokugawa jidai no yūmei na shin'i hōgen Ishizaka Sōtetsu" 徳川時代の有名な鍼医法眼石坂宗哲 [The famous "eyes of law" rank acupuncturist of the Tokugawa period Ishizaka Sōtetsu], *Jissen irigaku* 実践医理学 2: 1–5; 3: 355–371.

Lo, Vivienne 2005. "Quick and Easy Chinese Medicine: The Dunhuang Moxibustion Charts," in Vivienne Lo and Christopher Cullen, eds., *Medieval Chinese Medicine*. London: Routledge Curzon, 227–251.

Lu, Gwei-Djen, and Joseph Needham 2002. *Celestial Lancets: A History and Rationale of Acupuncture and Moxa*. London: Routledge Curzon.

Ma Jixing 馬継興 1993. *Zhenjiu tongren yu dongren xuefa* 鍼灸銅人与銅人穴法 [The acupuncture bronze figures and their acupuncture points]. Beijing: Zhongguo zhongyiyao chubanshe.

Macé, Mieko 1985. "La médecine à l'époque de Heian: Son organisation, son contenu théorique et ses rapports avec les courants de pensée contemporains." Ph.D. diss., University of Paris 7.

——— 1994a. "La médicine japonaise avant Meiji et la modernité," *Historiens et géographes* 344: 151–162.

——— 1994b. "The Medicine of Ishizaka Sōtetsu (1770–1841) as Cultural Pattern of the Edo Period: Based on the Example of Ei e chūkei zu (1825)," *Studia humana et naturalia* 28: 73–90.

Machi, Senjurō 町泉寿郎 2008. "Jūshikei hakki wo meguru shomondai: Nihon ni okeru juyō wo chūshin ni" 十四経発揮をめぐる諸問題—日本における受容を中心に [Some issues regarding the *Elucidations of the Fourteen Channels* focusing on its reception in Japan], *Keiraku chiryō* 経絡治療 174: 41–57.

Man'anpō 萬安方 (Formulas for Absolute Safety, 1327).

Manase Dōsan 曲直瀬道三 (1571) 1979a. *Keiteki shū* 啓迪集 [Compendium of the Keiteki]. *Kinsei kanpō igakusho shūsei* 近世漢方医学書集成 3. Tokyo: Meicho shuppan.

——— 1979b. *Kirigami* 切紙 [Paper strips]. *Kinsei kanpō igakusho shūsei* 近世漢方医学書集成 4. Tokyo: Meicho shuppan.

——— 1979c. *Shusshō haizai* 出証配剤 [Formulas given according to symptoms]. *Kinsei kanpō igakusho shūsei* 近世漢方医学書集成 4. Tokyo: Meicho shuppan.

——— 1995. *Shinkyū shūyō* 針灸集要 [Essentials of acupuncture and moxibustion]. *Manase Dōsan zenshū* 曲直瀬道三全集 2. Tokyo: Oriental shuppansha.

Mayanagi Makoto 真柳誠 2001. "Chūgoku iseki kiroku nendai sōmokuroku" 中国医籍記録年代総目録 [A general catalog of the dates of Chinese medical books recorded in Japanese sources], in Tadashi Yoshida 吉田忠 and Yasuaki Fukase 深瀬泰旦, eds., *Higashi to nishi no iryōbunka* 東と西の医療文化 [The medical culture of the East and West]. Kyoto: Shibunkaku shuppan, 17–51.

———— 2006. "Gendai Chūi shinkyūgaku no keisei ni ataeta Nihon no kōken" 現代中医鍼灸学の形成に与えた日本の貢献 [Japan's contribution to the establishment of modern Chinese acupuncture and moxibustion], *Zen Nihon shinkyū gakkai zasshi* 全日本鍼灸学会雑誌 56, 4: 605–615.

Mayanagi Makoto 真柳誠 and Tomobe Kazuhiro 友部和弘 1992. "Chūgoku iseki torai nendai mokuroku edoki" 中国医籍渡来年代総目録—江戸期 [A general catalog of the importation dates of Chinese medical books into Japan: Edo period], *Nihon kenkyū* 日本研究 7: 151–183.

Misono ie rekiden ryakki 御薗家歴伝略記 [A brief account of the history of the Misono family] 1989. *Kanpō zasshi fukkoku senshū* 漢方雑誌復刻選集 13. Osaka: Oriental shuppansha.

Murai Kinzan 村井琴山. *Idō nisennen ganmoku hen* 医道二千年眼目編 [Abbreviated volume of two thousand years of the way of medicine]. Waseda University Library (reference number: ya 09 00582).

Mushi no shirase: Kyūshū Kokuritsu Hakubutsukan zō Harikikigaki 虫の知らせ：九州国立博物館蔵「針聞書」 [Information on parasites: The *Account of Things Heard about Acupuncture* held by the Kyūshū National Museum] 2007. Tokyo: Jei Kyasuto.

Myōan Eisai 明菴栄西 (1211) 1994. *Kissa yōjōki* 喫茶養生記 [Notes on drinking tea to nourish life], in Furuta Shōkin 古田紹欽, ed., *Kōzen gokoku ron Kissayōjōki* 興禅護国論・喫茶養生記. Tokyo: Kōdansha.

Nagano Hitoshi 長野仁 2001a. *Hari kyū myujiiamu: Dōjinkei Meidōzu hen* はりきゅうミュージアム：銅人形・明堂図篇 [The Museum of Acupuncture and Moxibustion: Volume on bronze figures and Numinous Hall maps]. Osaka: Mori no miya iryo gakuen shuppanbu.

———— 2001b. "Kanbun kyū nensei Iimura Gensai kō dōjingyō oboegaki kishū wa wasei dōjingyō hasshō no chi ka" 寛文九年成・飯村玄斎考「銅人形」覚書—紀州は和製「銅人形」発祥の地か [Memorandum on bronze figures written by Iimura Gensai in *Kanbun* 9: Was Kishū the birthplace of Japanese bronze figures?], *Shinkyū Osaka* 鍼灸 17, 2: 5–8.

Nagano Hitoshi 長野仁 and Higashi Noboru 東昇 2007. *Sengoku jidai no hara no mushi: Hari kikigaki no yukai na byōma tachi* 戦国時代のハラノムシ：『針聞書』のゆかいな病魔たち [Parasites of the abdomen during the Sengoku period: The amusing demons of diseases in the *Account of Things Heard about Acupuncture*]. Tokyo: Kokushokan kōkai.

Nihonshoki 日本書紀 [Chronicles of Japan] (720) 1958. *Nihonkoten bungaku taikei* 日本古典文学大系 67–68. Tokyo: Iwanami shoten.

Peking chūigakuin hen 北京中医学院主編 1964. *Chūgoku igakushi kōgi* 中国医学史講義 [Lessons on the history of Chinese medicine], translated by Natsu Saburō 夏三郎. Tokyo: Ryōgen shoten.

Rhyne, Wilhelmi ten 1683. *Dissertatio de arthritide: Mantissa schematica; De acupunctura et orationes tres; I. De chymiae ac botaniae antiquitate & dignitate, II. De physiognomia, III. De monstris: singula ipsius authoris notis illustrator*. London: Impensis R. Chiswell.

Sano Midori 佐野みどり 1981. "Yamai no sōshi kenkyū" 病草紙研究 [Research on the *Scroll of Diseases*], *Kokka* 国華 1039: 7–28; 1040: 7–23.

Shindō hiketsu shū 鍼道秘訣集 [Compilation of secret methods related to the way of acupuncture] 1978. *Shinkyū igaku tenseki taikei* 鍼灸医学典籍大系 13. Tokyo: Shuppan kagaku sōgō kenkyūjo.

Shinohara Kōichi 篠原孝市 1994. "Ishinpō no shinkyū" 医心方の鍼灸 [Acupuncture and moxibustion in the *Formulas from the Heart of Medicine*], in *Ishinpō no kenkyū* 医心方の研究 [Research on *Formulas from the Heart of Medicine*]. Osaka: Oriental shuppansha, 99–120.

Shōsei Saidōtan 樵青斎洞丹 1994. *Enrashi shinkyū hō* 煙蘿子針灸法 [Enrashi's acupuncture and moxibustion methods], *Rinshō shinkyū keirakuketsusho shūsei* 臨床鍼灸経絡経穴書集成 58. Osaka: Oriental shuppansha.

Suganuma Shūkei 菅沼周圭 (1767) 1978. *Shinkyū soku* 鍼灸則 [Principles of acupuncture and moxibustion], *Shinkyū igaku tenseki taikei* 鍼灸医学典籍大系 17. Tokyo: Shuppan kagaku sōgō kenkyūjo.

Sun Simiao 孫思邈 (ca. 650–659) 1982. *Beiji qianjin yaofang* 備急千金要方 [Essential recipes for urgent use worth a thousand gold pieces]. Beijing: Renmin weisheng chubanshe yingyin.

Tanba no Yasuyori 丹波康頼 1991. *Ishinpō: Nakarai iemoto Ishinpō* 医心方: 半井家本 医心方 [Formulas from the heart of medicine: Edition of the Nakarai family]. Osaka: Oriental shuppansha.

Teramoto, John T. 1994. "The Yamai no sōshi: A Critical Reevaluation of Its Importance to Japanese Secular Painting of the Twelfth Century." Ph.D. diss., University of Michigan, Ann Arbor.

Tōryū i no gen'i 當流醫之源委 [On the origin of our school] 1777. Takeda kagaku shinkō zaidan kyōu shoya 武田科学振興財団杏雨書屋 (kan 乾 5445).

Unschuld, Paul 1995. "The Reception of Oriental Medicine in the West: Changing Worldview and Epistemological Adaptation," *Japanese Journal of Oriental Medicine* 45, 4: 745–754.

———— 2003. *Huang di nei jing su wen: Nature, Knowledge, Imagery in an Ancient Chinese Medical Text*. Berkeley: University of California Press.

Vigouroux, Mathias 2011. "Kinsei nihon ni okeru shinkyū no keisei to sono fukyū: Higashi ajia oyobi yōroppa no bunka kōryū no ichirei toshite" 近世日本における鍼灸医学の形成とその普及―東アジアおよびヨーロッパの文化交流の一例として [The making of Japanese acupuncture and its diffusion in early modern Japan as an example of the cultural interactions in East Asia and with Europe]. Ph.D. diss., Nishogakusha University, Tokyo.

Yakazu Dōmei 矢数道明 1982. *Kinsei kanpō igakushi: Manase Dōsan to sono gakutō* 近世漢方医学史—曲直瀬道三とその学統 [History of early modern *kanpō* medicine: Manase Dōsan and his family line]. Tokyo: Meicho shuppan.

Yamashina Tokitsune 山科言經 1959–1991. *Tokitsune kyōki* 言經卿記 [Tokitsune's diary]. Tōkyō Daigaku Shiryō Hensanjo hensan 東京大學史料編纂所編纂. Tokyo: Iwanami shoten.

Yōhō Takeshi 養老孟司 1995. "Igakubu hyōhonshitsu no hikari to kage" 医学部標本室の光と影 [Light and shadow of the specimen room of the faculty of medicine], *Geijutsu shinchō* 芸術新潮 15: 44–47.

Yu, Gengzhe 2007. "The Progression of Moxibustion Therapy in Tang and Song Dynasty Folk Medicine: An Analysis on the Background of Technology Choice," *Frontiers of History in China* 2, 3: 320–344.

Yūrin 有林 (ca. 1363) 1987. *Yūrin fukuden hō* 有林福田方 [Yūrin's Fukuden formulary]. Tokyo: Kagaku shoin.

CHAPTER 6

A Village Doctor and the *Treatise on Cold Damage Disorders* (*Shanghan lun* 傷寒論): Medical Theory / Medical Practice in Late Tokugawa Japan

Susan L. Burns

In recent years, studies of "village doctors" (*zaison'i* 在村医) have become an important topic for historians working on the social and cultural history of medicine in Tokugawa Japan (1600–1867). Some researchers have focused on the expansion of medical personnel and products, alerting us to the medicalization of health and illness beginning in the mid-eighteenth century as care by physicians and commodified medicinal products became available for the first time in rural areas where folk and faith-based practices had prevailed.[1] Others have explored the formation of regional and even countrywide networks of groups and individuals through which books and technology flowed, most notably those related to European medical knowledge such as anatomical texts and later smallpox vaccination.[2] A third strand of research has taken up the professionalization of physicians as a problem of the Tokugawa status system and explored the new cultural influence that some physicians enjoyed.[3] This essay aims to add to this literature by examining how medical knowledge took form at the village level, a topic with implications for all three of these issues. That is, it seeks to explore how a rural doctor who practiced far from Edo and Kyoto, the cities where elite medical professionals gathered, engaged with the canonical texts and the medical debates of his day. My goal is to consider, albeit in a preliminary way, the place of rural doctors within the medical culture of the late Tokugawa period.

To explore this issue, I will examine the work of the physician Nanayama Jundō 七山順道, who lived in the castle-town of Yūzawa in what is now Akita Prefecture in the first half of the nineteenth century. Born sometime around 1800, presumably in Yūzawa, Nanayama received his medical education in Kyoto, but he spent the entirety of his adult life practicing medicine in the villages

---

1   See, e.g., Tsukamoto 1986, 2001; Yamanaka 1994.
2   See, e.g., Aoki 1998. Also see the articles in Aoki 2004 and Hosono 2003.
3   Yokota 1996.

outside Yūzawa, one of several physicians active in this locality. The question of whether Nanayama was a "typical" village doctor is a knotty one. Certainly, he had scholarly aspirations. An enthusiastic bibliophile, he collected a substantial number of medical texts, more than sixty of which are still extant. Moreover, in the 1830s he began to compose works of his own, including two volumes of case notes and three works on the *Treatise on Cold Damage Disorders* (*Shanghan lun* 傷寒論; J. *Shōkanron*), a foundational text of the Chinese medical tradition that attracted significant attention from physician-scholars in eighteenth- and nineteenth-century Japan.[4] Although his book collecting and scholarly writing may have been distinctive, like other "village doctors" Nanayama never published any of his works, and I have not been able to identify him in any sources beyond those he authored. He viewed medicine as a family profession and seems to have written only for his own edification and that of his heirs. In an earlier essay, I examined Nanayama's case records and argued that they reveal the formation of a new medical consciousness that rigorously excluded magical medicine and folk practices.[5] In the present essay, in contrast, I explore Nanayama's commentaries on the *Treatise on Cold Damage Disorders*. I argue that through his engagement with the *Treatise*, Nanayama attempted to elucidate a foundation for his own practice, which relied on experimentation and observation.

Attributed to the Eastern Han physician Zhang Zhongjing 張仲景 (ca. 150–219 CE), the *Treatise on Cold Damage Disorders* is a clinical manual devoted to describing the origin, course, and treatment of externally contracted diseases termed collectively "Cold Damage disorders." Zhang's work is not extant, and the text as we know it today is said to be the work of Wang Shuhe 王叔和 (ca. 210–285 CE), who is believed to have substantially edited and reorganized the work. In its current form, the *Treatise on Cold Damage Disorders* describes six different disease patterns that result from exposure to cold, wind, and dampness and that are marked by different constellations of symptoms. These patterns are termed Greater Yang Disease, Yang Brightness Disease, Lesser Yang Disease, Greater Yin Disease, Lesser Yin Disease, Reverting Yin Disease. The *Treatise on Cold Damage Disorders* addresses treatment by delineating the specific formula necessary to treat each different combination of symptoms as they evolve during the course of an illness. For example, Greater Yang Disease, characterized by a floating pulse, stiffness and pain in the head and neck,

---

4   Nanayama's extant library, including his case notes and commentaries on the *Treatise on
      Cold Damage Disorders*, is held by the National Library of Medicine, Bethesda, Maryland.
      I am grateful to the staff of the library for their help during my visits.

5   Burns 2009.

aversion to cold, and fever, was to be treated by Cassia Twig Decoction 桂枝湯 (Ch. *gui zhi tang*, J. *keishitō*), while Lesser Yang Disease, characterized by fever, sweating, thirst, abdominal distention and pain, and constipation, called for the use of White Tiger Decoction 白虎湯 (Ch. *bai hu tang*, J. *hyakkotō*).[6] In total, the *Treatise on Cold Damage Disorders* contains 113 different formulas, using 72 different kinds of material medica.

In the Song period (960–1279), the first print version of the work appeared, and it soon became the object of sustained analysis by physician-scholars, who produced a large and complex body of commentary. In contrast, in Japan it was only in the seventeenth century that the *Treatise on Cold Damage Disorders* began to attract the attention of physicians. The most important figure in initially popularizing the text was the Kyoto-based physician Nagoya Gen'i 名古屋玄医 (1628–1696). In his 1679 work *Questions on Medical Treatments* (*Ihōmonyo* 医方問余), Nagoya famously paraphrased the *Treatise on Cold Damage Disorders* when he declared, "Of the myriad diseases, there is none that does not come from wind, cold, and dampness. If one wants to be specific and distinguish between them, one can speak of these three elements, but in general terms there is just the single one, cold."[7] Nagoya's enthusiasm for the *Treatise on Cold Damage Disorders* was shared by his contemporary Gotō Konzan 後藤艮山 (1659–1733), and together they are now considered the founders of the Ancient Formulas School (Koho-ha 古方派), which rejected the abstract diagnostic theorizing of post-Song medical theory that had been popularized in Japan by Manase Dōsan 曲直瀬道三 (1507–1594) and his students in the late sixteenth century, in favor of a pragmatic approach that focused on treatment and the alleviation of symptoms. With the coining of the term "Ancient Formulas," physicians who followed post-Song theories were (pejoratively, in many cases) termed the "latter-day school" (*gose-ha* 後世派). However, as Kosoto Hiroshi 小曽戸洋 has noted, the enthusiasm of Ancient Formulas physicians for the *Treatise on Cold Damage Disorders* did not mean that a new and coherent medical orthodoxy emerged: the complicated history of the *Treatise on Cold Damage Disorders* made it possible for physicians to valorize

---

6   For a summary of the history of the work and its contents, see Mitchell, Féng, and Wiseman 1999, 1–26. In translating the names of the formulas in the *Treatise on Cold Damage Disorders*, I have followed Mitchell, Féng, and Wiseman 1999, with the exception of that for 桂枝湯 (Ch. *gui zhi tang*, J. *keishitō*), which I translate as "Cassia Twig Decoction," following the translation used elsewhere in this volume. Mitchell, Féng, and Wiseman render this as "Cinnamon Twig Decoction."

7   Nagoya 1979, 5.

different aspects of the received text as "original" and to dismiss others as corrupt additions inserted by Wang Shuhe.[8]

By the time Nanayama Jundō traveled to Kyoto for medical training around 1818, the Ancient Formulas School was the dominant form of medical practice and the *Treatise on Cold Damage Disorders* boom was in full swing. Between 1770 and 1818, at least thirty commentaries on the *Treatise* were published, and others circulated in manuscript. These works took various forms. Most, such as Yamabe Bunhaku's 山辺文伯 *Annotated "Treatise on Cold Damage Disorders"* (*Shōkanron senchū* 傷寒論箋注, publ. 1779), drew upon both Japanese and Chinese commentaries and inserted annotations into the text, creating a dense network of references to other authors and other texts that was both a mode of argumentation and a display of scholarly credentials. But there were other approaches as well: as its title suggests, Ujiin Yōsaku's 雲林院了作 popular *A Japanese Account of the "Treatise on Cold Damage Disorders"* (*Shōkanron kokujikai* 傷寒論国字解, publ. 1771) offered an accessible summary of the text, while Hara Genrin's 原元麟 *A Graphic Explanation of the "Treatise on Cold Damage Disorders"* (*Shōkanron zusetsu* 傷寒論図説, publ. 1800) used a series of schematic diagrams to explain the work.[9]

Curiously, given his later interest in the *Treatise on Cold Damage Disorders*, Nanayama did not study with an Ancient Formulas physician, although there were many teaching in Kyoto at the time. For whatever reason, he entered the then-thriving school of Takenaka Fumisuke 竹中文輔 (1766–1836), known as the Seibidō 済美堂.[10] Takenaka himself had studied medicine with Wada Tōkaku 和田東郭, a representative figure of the so-called *setchūha* 折中派, or "syncretic school," that blended aspects of different approaches, including Ancient Formulas, post-Song, and so-called "Dutch medicine." Wada was a student of Yoshimasu Tōdō 吉益東洞 (1702–1773), a leading figure in Ancient Formulas circles, who is said to have declared that among the many ancient texts it was necessary to know only the *Treatise on Cold Damage Disorders* and the *Essential Prescriptions from the Golden Coffer* (*Jingui yaolue* 金匱要略),

---

8   Kosoto 1999, vii.

9   Kosoto provides an extremely useful survey of the Tokugawa period commentaries on the *Treatise on Cold Damage Disorders*; see Kosoto 1999, 185–214.

10   Evidence of Takenaka's reputation comes from 1813, 1822, and 1830 editions of the *Heian jinbutsu shi*, a "who's who" of Kyoto literati and scholars. See the searchable database of *Heian jinbutshu shi* hosted by the International Research Center for Japanese Studies: http://tois.nichibun.ac.jp/hsis/heian-jinbutsushi/Heian/index.html (accessed June 28, 2014).

another work attributed to Zhang Zhongjing.[11] Given this scholarly lineage, it is not surprising that Wada too was an admirer of the *Treatise on Cold Damage Disorders*: his students later edited his teachings into a work called *Understanding the Correct Text of the "Treatise on Cold Damage Disorders" (Shōkanron seibunkai* 傷寒論正文解, publ. 1844). But Wada eventually came to be an outspoken critic of both Yoshimasu's theory that "all diseases come from a single poison" and his reliance on harsh purgatives and emetics to expel the poison. Wada himself advocated a more nuanced approach to diagnosis and a gentler approach to treatment.[12] Nanayama was an admirer of Wada's work: he described his own discussion of the *Treatise on Cold Damage Disorders* formulas, entitled *Commentaries on the Ancient Formulas (Kohō ige* 古方意解), as based on his study of Wada's *Interpreting the Formulas (Hōikai* 方意解), an unpublished work that circulated only in manuscript.[13] It is unclear how long Nanayama studied with Takenaka or the content of his training, but it may have focused primarily on the preparation of herbal medicines. Only three works by Takenaka are extant, and all take the form of collections of formulas.

By 1824, Nanayama was back in Yūzawa and practicing medicine. Not long after his return, he began to compile notes on some of his patients, carefully documenting their symptoms and the course of treatment he offered them, focusing particularly on the effect of the medicines he prepared and prescribed, evidence perhaps of his training under Takenaka but also certainly of his engagement with the *Treatise on Cold Damage Disorders*. However, it was only in 1834 that Nanayama began to record his thoughts on the *Treatise*. In the preface that he attached to the work he called *Commentaries on the "Treatise on Cold Damage Disorders" (Shōkanron ige* 傷寒論意解), Nanayama described his motives: after he returned from Kyoto, he was so busy with his work that he had little time for scholarship until, in the autumn of 1834, he became severely ill for more than ten days and almost died. After his recovery, he felt it "a duty

---

11   Sakai 1982, 243. For a discussion of Yoshimasu's views of the *Yellow Emperor's Inner Canon* (*Huangdi neijing* 黃帝內經) and the *Divine Husbandman's Materia Medica* (*Shennong bencao jing* 神農本草經), see Tateno 2011, 5–8. On Yoshimasu, see also Daniel Trambaiolo's essay in the present volume.

12   Itō Takashi, "*Kanpō* ijin retsuden: Wada Tōkaku," *Tsumura medikaru tōdei*, http://medical. radionikkei.jp/tsumura/final/pdf/100526.pdf (accessed June 28, 2014).

13   Nanayama Jundō, *Shōkanron ige* (manuscript), vol. 1, 52–53. The manuscript has no page numbers. The page numbers used here and below reference my insertion of page numbers, counting from the first page of the main body of the text, after the prefaces. The preface by Nanayama Gen is dated 1868 and that by Nanayama Hiroshi is dated 1834. According to the *Union Catalogue of Early Japanese Books*, five copies of the *Hōikai* manuscript are extant.

of his occupation" to write up what he had learned for the benefit of his descendants and to aid "the course of day-to-day treatments" (*nichiyō chiryō no michi* 日用治療ノ道).[14] In short order he completed three works: *Commentaries on the "Treatise on Cold Damage Disorders," Commentaries on the Ancient Formulas*, and a second and far briefer discussion of the formulas called *On the Workings of the Ancient Formulas* (*Kohō kikatsu* 古方機活).

The rapid production of these works suggests that in the years following his return to Yūzawa, Nanayama was already immersed in studying the *Treatise on Cold Damage Disorders*. His extant library contains four commentaries on the work: *Collected Commentaries on the "Treatise on Cold Damage Disorders"* (*Shanghan lun ji zhu*; J. *Shōkanron shitchū*), by the famous Qing physician Gao Shishi 高世栻; *The Ancient Text of the "Treatise on Cold Damage Disorders"* (*Kobun Shōkanron* 古文傷寒論, publ. 1778), by Yoshimasu Tōdō and his student Momonoi Antei 桃井安貞; *The Definitive "Treatise on Cold Damage Disorders"* (*Shōkanron tsūdan* 傷寒論通斷, publ. 1795), by Shōji Juntai 東海林順泰; and *Famous Commentaries on the "Treatise on Cold Damage Disorders"* (*Shōkanron meigi* 傷寒論名義, manuscript), by Kawagoe Masayoshi 川越正淑.[15] Both the *Collected Commentaries on the "Treatise on Cold Damage Disorders"* and the *Famous Commentaries on the "Treatise on Cold Damage Disorders"* contain marginalia in Nanayama's hand, and the latter appears to have been transcribed by him as well—all evidence of his deep interest in the *Treatise on Cold Damage Disorders*.

But if Nanayama was well informed about the tradition of *Treatise* commentaries, he was also ultimately skeptical of their usefulness for a working physician like himself. The *Commentaries on the "Treatise on Cold Damage Disorders"* is his most sustained work on the *Treatise*. It consists of four volumes of commentary, each of about fifty pages, and addresses specific topics, such as the use of the pulses for diagnostic purposes, his experience with different disease patterns, and the efficacy of specific formulas for certain symptoms. Nanayama was overtly dismissive of both the Chinese and the Japanese tradition of commentaries. Chinese authors, he wrote, had failed to realize that the *Treatise on Cold Damage Disorders* was a critique of the *Yellow Emperor's Inner Canon* (*Huangdi neijing* 黄帝内經, composed between 400 BCE and 260 CE) and instead tried to understand it in light of the earlier work, a hermeneutic strategy that found textual expression when they inserted passages of the earlier text into their commentaries via interlineal annotations. According to Nanayama, by asserting the continuity of medical theory over time, they missed the

---

14   Nanayama, *Shōkanron ige*. Quotation is from the author's preface to vol. 1.

15   All these works are owned by the National Library of Medicine.

real significance of the *Treatise*—that it was a break with medical practice to that point. Many Japanese scholars too had misunderstood the work: the most egregious among them simply discarded portions of the text, most notably the discussion of the six patterns, although this, in Nanayama's view, was the important part of the work.

Needless to say, this is a problematic representation of the complex tradition of *Treatise* studies in both Japan and China, but Nanayama's claim that many Ancient Formulas physicians ignored the theoretical aspects of the *Treatise* in favor of its formulas is perceptive. In his recent work on *Treatise* studies in early modern Japan, Tateno Masami 舘野正美 has stated that Ancient Formulas doctors "used the *Treatise on Cold Damage Disorders* as a formulary" and ignored the six patterns.[16] Yoshimasu Tōdō, for one, took this approach in his famous *Categorized Formulas* (*Ruijūhō* 類聚方, publ. 1764), which in Keiko Daido's words, "deprived [the *Treatise*] of the pathological categorizations of three yin and yang and six channels," thus "enabling people to make prescriptions easily, even without an understanding of the systematic and theoretical formula-symptom correspondence that [the *Treatise*] contained."[17] Similarly, Endō Jirō 遠藤次郎 has argued that in putting forth his theory that "all diseases come from a single poison," Yoshimasu "rejected the three yang and three yin [patterns], the basic framework of [the *Treatise*]" and instead privileged the effects of the formulas described within it: vomiting, diarrhea, and sweating.[18]

The tendency of Ancient Formulas physicians to ignore the six patterns has thus been explained by referencing their concern for practice and disinterest in abstract theorizing. Nanayama too was deeply concerned with practice. He emphasized that his knowledge derived from his day-to-day practice of medicine (*hibi wagagyō to suru tokoro no michi* 日々我ガ業トスル所ノ道), not from "looking back" (*kaerimizu* 顧ズ) to early commentaries.[19] Reflecting this stance, the *Commentaries on the "Treatise on Cold Damage Disorders"* does not take the orthodox form of a commentary. Instead, Nanayama wrote in simple declarative language, in Japanese (*wabun* 和文) rather than classical Chinese (*kanbun* 漢文). But the work is not a rewriting of the *Treatise on Cold Damage Disorders* in Japanese like that produced by Ujiin Yōsaku and others. It assumes that its reader is already well versed in the content of the *Treatise* and provides a metacommentary that only occasionally engages with specific passages.

---

16   Tateno 2011, 4.
17   Daido, forthcoming.
18   Endō 2006, 163.
19   Nanayama, *Shōkanron ige*, vol. 1, 40–41.

But while Nanayama shared the concern for practice that ordered the Ancient Formulas approach to the *Treatise*, he distanced himself from many of his contemporaries in his concern for the six patterns, which he regarded as an essential aspect of the work. His *Commentaries* has two main themes—diagnostics and treatment—and Nanayama wrote that in regard to both the *Treatise* had been largely misunderstood by those who simply mined it for formulas. As he put it, "the point of the work is to explain how to treat the diseases of Cold Damage by dividing them into six patterns. This is the most important thing for treatment, and because Cold Damage is chief among all the myriad illnesses, you must know how to treat it."[20] In other words, the formulas could not be effectively utilized without understanding the theory behind them.

Nanayama was equally critical of those who misunderstood the patterns, treating them as a rigid set of stages that characterized the progression of every disease. He argued that rather than putting forth a doctrinaire approach to diagnosis and treatment, the *Treatise* in fact required physicians to be attentive to the individual variations of each patient's illness: "as for the course of a disease, people's bodies are different just as their faces are different. Therefore, the effects of the disease will not be the same."[21] Moreover, because the "transformation" (*tenpen* 転変) of Cold Damage is not fixed, it was impossible to predict the course of an illness.[22] For Nanayama then, the six patterns were a heuristic device that aided physicians in interpreting the multiple and often-evolving set of symptoms they observed, providing a foundation for treatment.

As this summary suggests, Nanayama was simultaneously dismissive of a reliance on purely textual knowledge and of a reductive approach to treatment in the name of practicality. Efficacious medical practice required not only an understanding of a body of medical theory but also an empirical knowledge of the workings of the individual body that could be derived only from sustained observation and practice. Nanayama's discussion of pulse diagnosis is similarly ordered by this perspective. Pulse diagnosis was the most important diagnostic tool within the *Treatise*, and Nanayama devoted a lengthy section of his *Commentaries* to this topic. He characterized the pulses as an important but difficult, and potentially unreliable, means by which to gauge the condition of a patient: "the theory is that since the pulse is the movement of the vital energy of the body, it should therefore reflect the other symptoms, but sometimes a patient can be near death and the pulses do not seem to accord with that; in other cases, the patient has no fever but if the apical pulse suddenly changes,

---

20   Ibid. 41–42.
21   Ibid., 43.
22   Ibid., 14. The term *tenpen* appears on p. 17.

then this is a bad symptom."[23] In other words, Nanayama suggested that a theoretical understanding of the pulses was insufficient to determine the condition of the patient, and he called upon practitioners to employ multiple diagnostic procedures. In his own case records, Nanayama not only typically took note of the pulses but also inspected the color and condition of the tongue, palpated the stomach, and observed the color and consistency of bodily waste.

In keeping with his concern for practice, Nanayama was critical of what he characterized as overly complex methods of pulse diagnosis, referring specifically to the twenty-four pulses that are described in Wang Shuhe's *Classic of Pulse Diagnosis* (*Maijing* 脈経). According to Nanayama, the discussion of twenty-four pulses "is extremely complex to explain and not especially helpful for treatment."[24] He noted that the *Treatise* makes mention of only eight different pulses and that these simply reflect three sets of qualities: rising or falling, slow or fast, slippery or knotty. Adopting the same line of argument he used in relation to the six patterns, Nanayama argued that the use of pulses for diagnostic purposes must also take note of individual variation: "the pulse depends upon the nature of each person, so each one is different. Even among the healthy, there are those who are strong and those who are weak. The strong may have fast and rising pulses, while the weak may have slow and falling pulses, so one should not generalize."[25] The physician's role then is to understand the pulse of the individual patient in question and to use its changes to understand the progress of the disease.

Nanayama's insistence that practice-based knowledge was more important than textual authority can be seen as well in his discussion of treatment. As I have already noted, the formulas of the *Treatise* were the most important aspect of the text for many Ancient Formulas physicians, and formularies had become an important form of medical writing. Yoshimasu Tōdō's *Categorized Formulas* was a groundbreaking text in this regard. Yoshimasu extracted 113 formulas from the *Treatise on Cold Damage Disorders* and the *Essential Prescriptions from the Golden Coffer* and organized them according to their main ingredient, bringing together, for example, all the formulas that had Cassia Twig as their primary ingredient. Each entry included information about the preparation and use of the formula, making the work an extremely useful handbook for physicians. The *Categorized Formulas* was phenomenally

---

23   Ibid., 46. The apical pulse (Ch. *xuli*, J. *kyuri*) was supposed to be palpable in the chest area and was generally believed to be a key indicator of the patient's condition.

24   Ibid., 44.

25   Ibid., 44–45.

successful: its first printing, said to be of ten thousand copies, sold out almost immediately, with the result that it was quickly reprinted and inspired many imitations.[26] However, Tateno has argued that in Yoshimasu's collection of fifty-three case records, *Notes on Special Cases* 建殊録 (*Kenshuroku*, publ. 1763), he only rarely made use of formulas from the *Treatise* in their received forms, choosing much more often to rely upon modified formulas or those from other, later sources. And this was by no means an approach peculiar to Yoshimasu.[27] Nakagami Kinkei 中神琴渓 (1744–1833), a student of Yoshimasu's and perhaps the most famous Ancient Formulas physician after Yoshimasu's death, declared the *Treatise on Cold Damage Disorders* to be the "compass, measure, and standard" (*kikujunjo* 規矩準縄) of medical care. Nonetheless, his case records reveal that he too rarely relied on its orthodox formulas.[28]

Like Yoshimasu and Nakagami, Nanayama also expressed reverence for the formulas of the *Treatise*, and he was critical of those who dismissed them as ineffective. He argued that the human body, like heaven and earth, was unchanged since antiquity and thus there was no basis for doubting the continuing efficacy of the formulas, if correctly used. According to Nanayama, if a formula appeared not to work, it was because the treating physician had failed to deploy it correctly: that is, he had not altered the formula according to the symptoms of his patient and his patient's particular constitution. In Nanayama's words, "now as in the past, it is necessary to adjust the different ingredients and the dosage on the basis of the symptoms, the severity of the illness, and the constitution of the patient. Thus, one cannot discuss treatment in indiscriminate terms, and you must always be extremely attentive to the change [in symptoms]."[29] What is important here is Nanayama's explicit claim that the *Treatise* itself authorized this kind of experimental approach: the formulas as recorded were always intended to be used as general guidelines that required modification by the physician.

In keeping with this valorization of the physician's skill and powers of observation, in his own study of the *Treatise* formulas, the *Commentaries on the Ancient Formulas*, Nanayama provided a detailed analysis of how the various ingredients in a specific formula influenced the body's workings both separately and in combination. Departing from the organizational strategy adopted by Yoshimasu in *Categorized Formulas*, which was widely emulated in other formularies, Nanayama did not list the formulas according to their primary

26   Kosoto 1999, 401.

27   Tateno 2011, 9.

28   Tateno 2011, 11.

29   Nanayama, *Shōkanron ige*, 3–4.

ingredient. Instead, the formulas are organized in a manner that seems designed to facilitate understanding of their relationship while illuminating the
effects of their differing ingredients. The work opens with a discussion of the
Cassia Twig Decoction, which Nanayama describes as the "founding father"
(*sogen* 祖元) of *Treatise* formulas. It consists of five ingredients: cassia twig,
white peony, fresh ginger, jujube dates, and fried licorice. According to Nanayama:

> In this formula the most important element is the cassia twig, the flavor
> of which is both sweet and hot. Its most important effect is to warm and
> to dissipate the damaging substance (*ja* 邪) that has penetrated the skin.
> It works by first warming the *ki* 気 (Ch. *qi*) of the stomach, which then
> moves [the damaging substance] to the outside of the skin so that it dis-
> sipates. Peony is sour and cold. Its most important effect is to settle in the
> kidneys, calm the *ki* of the stomach, and reduce the bodily fluids.... Gin-
> ger is hot. Its most important effect is to open up the mouth of the stom-
> ach so that stomach *ki* that produces phlegm is made to circulate. So it
> strengthens the effect of the cassia twig and helps expel the damaging
> substance that is moving out of the body.[30]

Nanayama concludes his discussion of the Cassia Twig Decoction by noting
that "both the formula and the symptoms are important. So you have to think
carefully and avoid treating the botanicals lightly."

A concern for explaining how simple additions and subtractions of ingredients change the effects of a formula is the organizing motif of the *Commentaries on the Ancient Formulas*. Following this extended discussion of the Cassia
Twig Decoction, Nanayama turns next to the formula known as Minor Center
Fortifying Decoction (Ch. *xiao jian zhong tang* 小建中湯, J. *shōkenchūtō*). It
consists of the same five ingredients as the Cassia Twig Decoction with the
addition of malt sugar and increases in the amounts of peony and licorice.
According to Nanayama, the change in the ingredients and their proportions
means that the formula has an entirely different effect: "the Center Fortifying Decoction works inwardly, while the Cassia Twig Decoction's action is
outwardly. And the most important ingredient in the Center Fortifying Decoction is the white peony, and the additional licorice combines with the peony in

---

30   Nanayama Jundō, *Keihō ige* 経方意解 (*Commentaries on the Ancient Formulas*). Manu-
      script held by the National Library of Medicine. This copy dates from 1868. The text has no
      page numbers, but the quotation is from the first two pages of the body of the work, fol-
      lowing the table of contents.

order to sooth the stomach and make it loose." The next formula to be discussed is the Pueraria Decoction (Ch. *gegen tang* 葛根湯, J. *kakkontō*), which
consists of the same five ingredients as the Cassia Twig Decoction plus ephedra and kudzu. Now the two new ingredients become the most important
within the formula: both promote sweating, a means to expel the damaging
forces of Wind and Cold.

The rest of the work continues in this manner, explaining the relationship
of one formula to another and the workings of their ingredients. Clearly, the
Commentaries on the Ancient Formulas was not a simple "handbook" that
matched formula to symptom. It was a treatise on formula making that reflected Nanayama's efforts to understand the effects of the botanicals, singu-
larly and in combination. His explanations appear to have been based upon
Nanayama's experience in treating his own patients. His case notes meticulously recorded the course of his patients' illnesses and the treatments he provided. An example is the care he provided to a fifteen-year-old girl named
Tsume in the eighth month of 1827.[31] Nanayama initially observed that she had
a headache, fever and chills, stomach pain, and constipation, that her tongue
had a yellow coating and black spots, that her skin was burning hot, and that
she had a hard lump in the left side of her chest. He concluded that she was
suffering from *jieki* 時疫, a term applied to a seasonal epidemic disease characterized by high fever that may have been typhoid fever.

To treat Tsume, Nanayama first used the Major Bupleurum Decoction (Ch.
da chai hu tang 大柴胡湯, J. *daisaikotō*). The patient's stomach pains eased, as
did her constipation, but her fever continued and she became delirious.
Nanayama responded by dosing her with the Minor Bupleurum Decoction
(Ch. *xiao chai hu tang* 小柴胡湯, J. *shōsaikotō*) in combination with the Coptis
Decoction (J. *ōrentō* 黄蓮湯), to which he added bamboo shavings (*chikujo* 竹
茹) and gypsum (*sekkō* 石膏). Ten days passed and his patient's condition continued to decline. Her pulse was irregular; her tongue and lips were black; her
breathing was labored; and her belly was distended and painful. Nanayama
speculated that a "bad *ki*" had entered her stomach and that the fever was at its
peak. He responded with the Major Qi Coordinating Decoction (Ch. *da cheng
qi tang* 大承氣湯, J. *daijōkitō*). Several days later, his patient developed a red
rash that spread over her body. Nanayama gave her another dose of the Major
Qi Coordinating Decoction but followed it with White Tiger Decoction. Finally,
Tsume's fever fell, but she was still very ill, and Nanayama believed that the

---

31   Nanayama Jundō, *Nanzandō chiken* 南山堂治験 (*Case Records of the Nanzandō*), vol. 1,
      case 107. Manuscript held by the National Library of Medicine. This copy dates from 1868.
      The pages are not numbered. The case numbers are my own.

disease was now progressing internally. He again prescribed the Major Qi Co-ordinating Decoction but followed it with Bamboo Shaving Warm the Liver Decoction (Ch. *zhu ru wen dan tang* 竹茹温胆湯, J. *chikujō ontantō*), to which he added gypsum. The girl's fever again fell but her pulse was slow, and her tongue was bright red with a large half-moon-shaped crack in its center. Nanayama tried one final medicine, Raise the Yang and Dispel the Fire Decoc-tion (Ch. *sheng yang san huo tang* 升陽散火湯, J. *shōyōsankatō*), but it was no use. Thirty-five days after he had first examined her, Tsume died.

Scholar-physicians in this period—those with ties to important medical lin-eages who wrote and published commentaries, case notes, and formularies—often disparaged the skills of ordinary practitioners, who they asserted turned to medical practice out of a desire for profit and who lacked training, skill, and moral character. The prolonged suffering and eventual death of Tsume might be viewed as evidence of Nanayama's lack of skill, although even today as many as 30 percent of those infected with typhoid fever will die unless treated with modern antibiotics. But the real significance of Nanayama Jundō's work as re-corded in his case notes and commentaries lies beyond the fate of any single patient. Taken together, his writings and library reveal the emergence and ex-pansion of a new episteme of medical knowledge in which expertise gained from observation, experience, and experimentation was increasingly valued over text-based knowledge. This did not mean that texts were irrelevant: as we've seen, the *Treatise on Cold Damage Disorders* emerged as an important locus of medical discourse, allowing for debate, dissent, and the articulation of new approaches. Tateno has described the work as a "symbol" for Ancient For-mulas practitioners. To a degree, he is correct: the *Treatise* was used to promote a new ethos of practical knowledge through the culturally authorized concep-tion of "returning to ancient ways."[32] But it was more than that as well. As we have seen from Nanayama's work, the *Treatise* was also a powerful catalyst for innovation. He approached it not as a canonical work, in the traditional sense of that word, but rather as an exemplification of a methodology by which to approach diagnosis and treatment.

The new episteme was as much a social as an intellectual formation. Both the flourishing print culture and the emergence of Kyoto as a site of profes-sional training for would-be physicians from all over the country made it pos-sible for Nanayama, an ordinary resident of a small provincial town far from the cultural centers of early modern Japan, to participate in the most pressing medical debates of his time. Significant as well were the new "medical market-places" forming at the level of town and village, in which multiple physicians

---

32   Tateno 2011, 11.

vied with each other for patients. By the 1820s the residents of Yūzawa and the nearby villages, like those in many other regions in Japan, had available to them the services of multiple physicians. Nanayama's case records reveal that he was in constant competition with other doctors, whom he replaced or who replaced him, as patients and their families sought better, faster results.[33] For many consumers within this new medical landscape, effective treatments were no doubt more important than scholarly credentials or intellectual lineage, and so physicians needed to master new skills and pursue new treatments. As a result, a reputation for skill, as well as medical knowledge, became a crucial constituent of professional identity.

References

Aoki Toshiyuki 青木歳幸. 1998. *Zaison rangaku no kenkyū* 在村蘭学の研究 [Research on Dutch Learning at the village level]. Kyoto: Shibunkaku shuppan.

——— 2004. "Chiiki rangaku no sōgōteki kenkyū" 地域蘭学の総合的研究 [Comprehensive research on Dutch Learning at the local level. Special issue of *Kokuritsu minzoku hakubutsukan kenkyū hōkoku* 国立民族博物館研究報告116 (March).

Burns, Susan L. 2009. "Nanayama Jundō at Work: A Village Doctor and Medical Knowledge in Early Modern Japan." *East Asian Science, Technology, and Medicine* 29: 62–83.

Daido, Keiko (forthcoming). "The Reconstruction of the *Treatise on Cold Damage* in Eighteenth Century Japan: Text, Society, and Readers." *Asian Medicine: Tradition and Modernity*.

Endō Jirō 遠藤次郎 et al. 2006. *Iyasu chikara wo saguru: Higashi no igaku to nishi no igaku* 癒す力をさぐる：東の医学と西の医学 [Exploring the power to heal: Medicine in the East and medicine in the West]. Tokyo: Nōsangyoson Bunka Kyōkai.

Hosono Kentarō 細野健太郎 2003. "Iryō ni miru mura shakai to Edo: Ishikan no kōryū wo chūshin ni" 医療にみる村社会と江戸:医師間の交流を中心に [Village society and Edo as seen in medicine: With a focus on the interaction of physicians], in Takeuchi Makoto 竹内誠, ed., *Tokugawa bakufu to kyodai toshi Edo* 徳川幕府戸巨大都市江戸 [The Tokugawa *bakufu* and the great city Edo]. Tokyo: Tōkyōdō shuppan, 417–446.

Kosoto Hiroshi 小曽戸洋 1999. *Nihon kanpō tenseki jiten* 日本漢方典籍辞典 [A dictionary of Japan's Sino-Japanese medical texts]. Tokyo: Taishukan Shoten.

Mitchell, Craig, Féng Yè, and Nigel Wiseman. 1999. *Shāng Hán Lùn: On Cold Damage; Translation and Commentaries.* Brookline, MA: Paradigm.

---

33   Nagata 2004 addresses the issue of physician choice.

Nagata Naoko 長田直子 2004. "Kinsei kōki ni okeru kanja no ishi sentaku: 'Suzuki Heikyūrō kōshi nikki' wo chūshin ni" 近世後期における患者の医師選択—『鈴木平九郎公私日記』を中心に [How did patients choose a doctor in the late Tokugawa period? With a focus on the journal of Suzuki Heikyūrō], *Kokuritsu minzoku hakubutsukan kenkyū hōkoku* 国立民族博物館研究報告 116 (March): 317–341.

Nagoya Gen'i 名古屋玄医 1979. "*Ihōmonyo*" 医方問余 [Questions on medical treatments], in Ōtsuka Keisetsu 大塚敬節 et al., eds., *Kinsei kanpō igakusho shūsei* 近世漢方医学書集成 [An anthology of early modern Sino-Japanese medical texts], vol. 102. Tokyo: Meichō shuppan, 8–215.

Sakai Shizu 酒井シヅ 1982. *Nihon no iryōshi* 日本の医療史 [A history of Japanese medicine]. Tokyo: Tokyo Shoseki.

Tateno Masami 館野正美 2011. "Edo jidai no koihō no igaku to *Shōkanron*: Edo jidai no igaku no issokumen" 江戸時代古医方の医学と『傷寒論』：江戸時代医療の一側面 [Ancient Formulas medicine and the *Treatise on cold damage disorders* in the Edo period: One aspect of Edo period medicine], *Seikatsu bunkashi* 生活文化史 60: 3–17.

Tsukamoto Manabu 塚本学 1986. "Minzoku no henka to kenryoku—Kinsei Nihon no iryō ni okeru" 民族の変化と権力 [Power and the transformation of folk life: Medicine in early modern Japan], in *Kinsei saikō* 近世再 [Rethinking early modern Japan]. Tokyo: Nihon Edetā Skūru, 149–176.

——— 2001. *Ikirukoto no kinseishi* 生きることの近世史 [A history of living in early modern Japan]. Tokyo: Heibonsha.

Yamanaka Hiroyuki 山中浩之 1994. "Zaigōmachi no okeru ika to iryō no tenkai" 在郷町における医家と医療の展開 [The development of doctors and medical treatments in rural towns], in Nakabe Yoshiko 中部よしこ, ed., *Ōsaka to shūhen shotoshi no kenkyū* 大阪と周辺諸都市の研究 [Research on Osaka and nearby cities]. Osaka: Seibundō shuppan, 369–443.

Yokota Fuyuhiko 横田冬彦 1996. "Kinsei minshū shakai ni okeru chiteki dokusho no seiritsu" 近世民衆社会における知的読書の成立 [The rise of scholarly reading among early modern commoners], *Edo no shisō* 江戸の思想 5: 48–67.

Honzōgaku after *Seibutsugaku*: Traditional Pharmacology as Antiquarianism after the Institutionalization of Modern Biology in Early Meiji Japan

Federico Marcon

The Meiji Restoration (*Meiji ishin* 明治維新) of 1868 marked the beginning of a process of radical modernization that transformed Japan into a nation-state with vibrant intellectual and scientific communities, a growing capitalist economy, a strong army, and a rich colonial empire. And yet, the events of 1868 were too anticlimactic to be called revolutionary. Life for the majority of the population continued unchanged in the months following the collapse of the Tokugawa *bakufu* 徳川幕府, and the political elites at the local level remained in power as administrators of their lands as before. The Meiji Restoration of 1868 may not qualify to be considered a revolution comparable to the American or the French of the late eighteenth century, but the changes that occurred between the 1850s and the 1880s transformed Japanese society so radically that describing them as revolutionary would not be an exaggeration: a revolution in the *long durée*. The persistence of the trope of "change and continuity" in the historiography of modernizing Japan is evidence of the ostensible contradictions of revolutionary changes after an *un*revolutionary event.

A different approach to the unfolding of the Meiji "revolution" in the second half of the nineteenth century follows the transformation of traditional cultural fields in the early decades of the Meiji period. Many literary and artistic styles and genres, as well as fields of knowledge, disappeared; others changed and adapted under the pressure of new ideas and new forms introduced from the West. In the following pages, I reconstruct the processes through which a field of nature study that developed in the Tokugawa period out of a corpus of Chinese medicinal texts in the Confucian tradition—known under the umbrella term of *honzōgaku* 本草学—was adapted and transformed into the modern fields of biology (*seibutsugaku* 生物学), botany (*shokubutsugaku* 植物学), and zoology (*dōbutsugaku* 動物学) in the 1870s and 1880s.

In the course of the Tokugawa period, the discipline of *honzōgaku*—literally "the study of the fundamental herbs," a field of pharmacological research ancillary to medical studies—developed into an eclectic field of nature studies that encompassed an array of styles and approaches, from lexicography and encyclopedism to agronomy, aesthetics, gastronomy, and natural history. These *exaptive* transformations resulted from radical shifts in the standards, practices, and socio-professional configurations that characterized the study of the natural world, such that a primarily lexicographic discipline could become an empirical science that was surprisingly easily assimilated into the modern Meiji state in the second half of the nineteenth century.[1] A combination of intellectual, social, political, aesthetic, and economic changes made the new forms of natural knowledge possible: above all, the development of a market economy, improvements in agricultural production, mercantilist policies of shogunal and domainal administrations, and increased exchange of cultural goods across different social classes—an exchange that favored a surge of popular entertainment, refined pastimes, artistic creations, and intellectual discourse related to plants and animals.[2] Concerns with economic necessity and educated entertainment dominated these transformations and contributed to produce a discipline (or, better put, an ensemble of disciplines and practices) that accumulated an impressive load of data on plants and animals, as well as a sophisticated technology of observation, description, reproduction, and manipulation of specimens.

Toward the end of the Tokugawa period, however, the rich diversity of styles, approaches, forms, and ends of Japanese *honzōgaku* gave way to a more integrated discipline, the instrumental value of which was mobilized for the sake of economic growth. Three factors contributed to this process of simplification: deep fractures in the social texture that the monetized and market-oriented economy stimulated; the economic crisis of the 1830s, which called for a complete reformation of both the political sphere and the productive system; and the acceptance of the new Western sciences by a larger number of scholars and naturalists, thanks to the activities of the German physician and

---

1   "Exaptation" is a term I adopted from evolutionary biology. It was used by Stephen Jay Gould in 1982 to refer to a shift in the function of a trait or feature that was not produced by natural selection for its current use. Perhaps the feature was produced by natural selection for a function other than the one it currently performs and was then co-opted for its current function. For example, feathers might have originally arisen in the context of selection for insulation, and only later were they co-opted for flight. In this case, the general form of feathers is an adaptation for insulation and an exaptation for flight. See Gould and Vrba 1982.

2   Marcon, forthcoming; Nishimura 1999.

botanist Franz von Siebold, surgeon at the Dutch East Indies station of Deshima, in Nagasaki Bay.

After the Tenpō 天保 crisis of the 1830s, the instrumental value of *honzōgaku* for economic growth became a leading impulse for its practices. This transformation in scopes and methods put in motion two distinct but interrelated dynamics. On the one hand, *honzōgaku* became more similar to Western natural history, in particular that brand of naturalistic research sponsored by Linnaeus and his "apostles," which submitted natural knowledge to the necessities of national economic growth.[3] On the other hand, I claim that the fusing of *honzōgaku* and the new field of *keizaigaku* 経済学—a Confucian notion translatable as "ordering the realm and saving the people" that soon transformed into "political economy"—facilitated the conversion of late Tokugawa scholars into modern scientists in the early decades of the Meiji period.[4]

After the defeat of the Tokugawa and their allies in the Boshin War 戊辰戦争 (1868–1869) and the founding of a new political system that restored power to the emperor, Japanese politicians and scholars engaged in a modernization effort that lasted for at least the first three decades of the Meiji period. Amnesia and erasure of the recent Tokugawa past were a vital prerequisite of this endeavor of "civilizing and enlightening" (*bunmei kaika* 文明開化) Japan and the Japanese.[5] At the same time, the manufacturing of its national subjects involved the canonization (which often coincided with its invention) of a "national literature," a "national history," a "national religion," and a "national language."[6]

A different attitude characterized the political, financial, and intellectual endorsement of those disciplines—most importantly, the various scientific disciplines—that were "adopted" from the West and were fundamental for laying the industrial and economic foundations of the new nation-state. James Bartholomew well summarized the dominant attitude of Meiji scholars and statesmen, for whom "[t]he paradigms in effect in the Tokugawa period were all replaced by Western ones, and government policies restricting certain fields did not survive the demise of the shogunate."[7] In actual fact, if we follow the fate of *honzōgaku* in the transition from the Tokugawa to the Meiji period, a more complex and nuanced picture emerges. On the one hand, *honzōgaku* lost its name and transferred to the practitioners of the new scientific fields two

3   Koerner 2001.

4   Fujita 2003.

5   Gluck 1985; Shimane Kenritsu Daigaku Nishi Amane Kenkyūkai 2005; Kōsaka 1999.

6   Narita 2002.

7   Bartholomew 1989, 9.

centuries of knowledge, research, data, images, techniques, attitudes, styles, facilities, expertise, schools, social relations, books, embalmed and dried specimens, and so on. Scholars active in the transitional period of the 1850s to the 1880s were able to translate Western taxonomy and observational procedures into the familiar language of *honzōgaku*, so that the terminology developed in the Tokugawa period was adapted to convey Western concepts. On the other hand, *honzōgaku* became the name—associated with *kanpōyaku* 漢方藥, now referring to *traditional* (Chinese) medicine in antagonistic opposition to Western medicine—of a lost tradition, of a forgotten wisdom, of alternative practices, of a repository of Asian identity.

A glance at the names and biographies of some of the best-known scientists active in the first half of the Meiji period shows that, at least in the natural sciences, the Meiji Restoration brought more continuity than rupture. Mori Risshi 森立之, a physician of the Fukuyama domain 福山藩 and a strong advocate of the restoration of classical Chinese *honzōgaku*, became a high-ranking bureaucrat in the Ministry of Finance (1869) and the Ministry of Education (1871) with responsibility for scientific education.[8] Yamamoto Keigu 山本溪愚, whose father, Yamamoto Bōyō 山本亡羊, was a direct disciple of the famous *honzōgaku* scholar Ono Ranzan 小野蘭山, continued his father's activity in his private school in Osaka and spent his time organizing meetings that were regularly attended by both *honzōgaku* amateurs and Japanese biologists.[9] Ono Motoyoshi 小野職愨, son of Ono Ranzan's nephew Ono Mototaka 小野蕙畝, was another high-ranking bureaucrat in the Ministry of Education.[10] He was responsible, together with Tanaka Yoshio 田中芳男, for the administration and activities of the Office of Natural History, the Hakubutsukyoku 博物局. The office was established in the ninth month of 1871 as a substitute for the shogunal Office of Products (Bussankyoku 物産局) and acted as an interministerial agency connecting the Ministry of Education with the Ministry of Agriculture and Commerce and the Home Ministry, coordinating the collaboration of natural scientists with the government. Its first act was the establishment of the Tokyo National Museum of Natural History. Tanaka Yoshio, one of Itō Keisuke's 伊藤圭介 many students, was one of its founders. Tashiro Yasusada 田代安定, a pioneer in the study of East Asian tropical vegetation, received a formal education in *honzōgaku* in the Satsuma domain 薩摩藩 before he became a member of the Office of Natural History at the

---

8   In Japanese, *kohonzō fukko*. Ueno 1991, 138–144.

9   Ueno 1991, 145–148.

10   Ueno 1991, 148–151. Ono Mototaka was a member of the shogunal Institute of Medicine (Igakukan 医学館).

Ministry of Education after the Restoration.[11] When the University of Tokyo was founded in 1877, of the fifteen tenured professors in the new Department of Science, twelve were foreigners and the remaining three consisted of a professor of botany, Yatabe Ryōkichi 矢田部良吉, a professor of applied mathematics, Kikuchi Dairoku 菊池大麓, and a professor of metallurgy, Imai Iwao 今井巌, all of whom began their education in *honzōgaku* and Neo-Confucian studies in domainal schools and specialized, after 1868, in Western studies with periods of research abroad.

The composition of the early faculty of the science departments of the University of Tokyo reflected, in both style and method, the way science was being studied and taught in the West. Itō Keisuke was the scholar who inspired the first generation of Japanese natural scientists after his employment as adjunct professor shortly after the university was founded. This founding scientific generation included Iijima Isao 飯島魁, son of a retainer of the Hamamatsu domain 浜松藩, who graduated from the University of Tokyo under Itō Keisuke's supervision and became a pioneering zoologist.[12] The same was true for Miyoshi Manabu 三好学, a botanist born in a samurai family of the Noto domain 能登藩.[13] Another notable figure was the botanist Shirai Mitsutarō 白井光太郎, whose graduating dissertation was highly praised by his adviser, Itō Keisuke, and who would become one of the first modern historians of *honzōgaku*.[14]

Both the social origins and the worldviews of Meiji natural scientists were more similar to the ones held by *honzōgaku* scholars before 1868 than the conventional historical narratives suggest. Tokugawa research practices were not abandoned, and the rise of modern natural sciences in Meiji Japan is better described as a slow transformation and adaptation of *honzōgaku* practices and theories to the language, methods, and aims of Western sciences. The classification of plants and animals changed as the scientific taxonomy derived from Linnaeus replaced the divisions established by Li Shizhen's 李時珍 *Bencao gangmu* 本草綱目 (*Systematic Materia Medica*; *Honzō kōmoku* in Japanese). But the severity of this disruption was mitigated by the use of *honzōgaku* terminology to convey Western-derived biological concepts. For example, the names of the taxonomical divisions of the *Bencao gangmu* were carried over as the names of genera, families, orders, and classes of biological systematics. Chemistry and cellular biology coexisted with natural history (*hakubutsugaku*

---

11   Ueno 1991, 169–176.

12   Ueno 1991, 180–189.

13   Ueno 1991, 190–196.

14   Ueno 1991, 197.

博物学), which was still concerned with classification and fieldwork activities resembling *honzōgaku* herbalist expeditions.[15]

This uniformity in attitudes was in part the result of the socially homogeneous background of the first Japanese scientists. Like their *honzōgaku* predecessors, they understood natural studies as a form of service for the welfare of the state. The majority of them collaborated with the Office of Natural History either as organizers of science curricula in the new national education system or as consultants in the development of agricultural reform and industrial planning.[16] The activities of Tanaka Yoshio, Itō Keisuke's student both before and after the Meiji Restoration, exemplify the connection between natural history and the government. He was one of the founders of the interministerial Office of Natural History in 1870, of both the Ueno Zoological Garden and the first Museum of Natural History of Japan (1873), and of the Agricultural Association of Great Japan (1881).[17]

Tanaka was a scholar involved in various public activities, but even more research-oriented scientists like Shirai Mitsutarō could not avoid contacts with governmental offices. After his graduation from the Imperial University in 1886, Shirai found employment as lecturer, thanks to Tanaka's recommendation, in the Tokyo School for Agricultural and Forest Studies (Tokyo nōrin gakkō 東京農林学校), administered by the Ministry of Agriculture and Commerce. After the school was annexed to the Imperial University in 1893 as the Department of Agriculture, Shirai became an associate professor there. For the remainder of his career, he was involved in survey programs organized by the Ministry of Agriculture in various regions of the country. He is remembered today as the first historian of Japanese traditional natural history, but also for having authored a number of works on Japanese forests, his favorite being a survey of Japanese trees he entitled *Jumoku wamyō kō* 樹木和名考 (*Reflections on the Japanese Names of Trees*, published posthumously in 1933). This text was conceived and written in perfect *honzōgaku* style—as the title itself suggests.[18] Shirai summarized his decades of field expeditions sponsored by the Ministry of Agriculture, providing a list of the various regional names of each tree and giving information on its utilization in the Tokugawa period and how it could contribute to the economic growth of the nation. The text was

---

15   Prince Hachisuka Masauji 蜂須賀正氏 continued the tradition of *honzōgaku* patronage by taking part in naturalist expeditions in Africa and Southeast Asian regions, including Taiwan. See Hachisuka 2006; Kagaku 1991.

16   Nishimura 1999, 2:520–527, 544–556.

17   Miller 2013.

18   Shirai 1933.

written in the classical Japanese style used to translate Chinese throughout the Tokugawa period (*kundoku kakikudashi* 訓読書下) and is indistinguishable from an early modern *honzōgaku* text, except for the scientific Latin name attached to each species.

Hence, *honzōgaku*, as a name for natural studies, disappeared in the Meiji period, but in part it survived in form and content under the new rubric of *hakubutsugaku*, "natural history." Tokugawa scholars, called *jusha* 儒者, also disappeared. Yet their successors shared many of their inclinations, not least of which being the call to public service, though they were now known either by their professional titles or generically as *gakusha* 学者 or *shikisha* 識者, simply "scholars," terms that had begun to circulate only toward the end of Tokugawa period, or as *hakase* 博士, "scientists," a term adopted from the old imperial school of the Daigakuryō 大学寮 of seventh-century Japan. Just as the *honzōgaku* spirit survived in modern *hakubutsugaku*, the social role of scholar-officials, of Tokugawa *jusha*, continued to characterize the life of many intellectuals in modern Japan. As Andrew Barshay put it, "the vector of national service was very powerful; thinkers who were internally alienated could often be restored to the national community."[19] Many scientists were enlisted by the Meiji government in the service of modernization and directed their research activity to that purpose. They were now called biologists, botanists, and zoologists, but their scholarly activities resembled those of their Tokugawa predecessors. This passage from *honzōgaku* to *hakubutsugaku*—just like the passage from *jusha* to *gakusha* or *hakase*—in the Meiji period suggests that although the names of the discipline and its practitioners changed, the Tokugawa legacy lived on and informed the modern names of nature.

At the same time and parallel to these developments, *honzōgaku* kept its name in explicitly antagonistic opposition to the modernization of medicine. This meant opposition to rapid institutional changes that privileged Western medicine and marginalized traditional medicine, as well as opposition to the rapid disavowal of the intellectual legacies of the Tokugawa period upon which *honzōgaku* was founded.

To understand the dynamic of the survival of the term *honzōgaku* when associated with traditional medicine, it is first of all worth briefly sketching the development of medical-training institutions in nineteenth-century Japan. In 1858 the private school Shutōsho 種痘所 was founded in Edo to cure smallpox and was modeled upon the Nagasaki 長崎 clinic run by Otto Gottlieb Mohnike since 1849. Two years later, in 1860, the Shutōsho merged with the educational facilities of the shogunate and, together with the Institute of Medicine

---

19   Barshay 2004, 241. See also Gluck 1985.

(Igakukan), became the central institution for the study of Western medicine, under the name of the School of Medicine (Igakkō 医学校, 1863). After the Meiji Restoration, the School of Medicine was united in a sort of corporation with the former Hayashi 林 school of Zhu Xi studies 朱子学 (the Shōheikō 昌平校) and with the shogunal professional school, Kaiseigakkō 開成学校, and beginning in 1869 they became known, respectively, as University Eastern School (Daigaku tōkō 大学東校), University (Daigaku 大学), and University Southern School (Daigaku nankō 大学南校). The University Eastern School, at first under the supervision of the British physician William Willis, since its beginning had strong ties with the Military Hospital of Yokohama 横浜. In 1871 the German physicians Leopold Müller and Theodor Hoffmann became the leading instructors at the school. In 1874 it was renamed Tokyo Medical School (Tokyo Igakkō) and became the main medical-training center in early Meiji Japan: the majority of the first generation of its Japanese students were physicians formerly educated in Chinese medicine. From 1872 to 1875 the faculty of the Tokyo Medical School expanded to include the German physicians von Baelz, Niewerth, Martin, Langgaard, Korschelt, and Hansen in order to cope with the growing number of enrolling students.

It was in the context of this rapid development of a modern Japanese field of Western medicine that the activities of Asada Sōhaku 浅田宗伯 (1815–1894), physician of traditional Chinese medicine, became renowned in the modern city of Tokyo. A former student of Rai San'yō 頼山陽, Asada had studied Chinese medicine with Taki Motokata 多紀元堅, Kojima Naokata 小島尚質, and Kitamura Naohiro 喜田村直寛, all physicians of the shogunal Institute of Medicine. Today, Asada Sōhaku is probably most remembered as the inventor of the recipe for the Asada *ame* 浅田飴, better known as *nodoame* 喉飴, candies that help to alleviate the symptoms of sore throats that we can still buy in every convenience store in Japan. But in the early Meiji period, in the context of rapid Westernization and modernization, Asada was a living relic of a disappearing world or, better put, a world in the process of being disavowed and erased. Natsume Sōseki 夏目漱石, in his 1906 *Wagahai wa neko dearu* 我が輩は猫である (*I Am A Cat*), has offered a revealing portrait of Asada:

> Now, there flourished in the days of my master's childhood a certain noted physician of Chinese medicine, Asada Sōhaku, who lived in Ushigome. When that old man went out upon his rounds, he invariably traveled, very, very slowly, in a palanquin. As soon as he was dead, and his adopted son had taken over the practice, the palanquin was put away in favor of a rickshaw. No doubt in time's due course the adopted son's

adopted son will put away the invariable herb tea of his predecessors and start prescribing aspirin; however, even in the first Sōhaku's heyday, it was regarded as shabbily old-fashioned to be troudled through the streets of Tokyo in a palanquin. Only long established ghosts, dead pigs on their way to freight yards, and, of course, Sōhaku's doddering self saw nothing unpresentable about it.[20]

Asada, this "shabbily old-fashioned" physician of *kanpōyaku*, must have appeared as an anachronistic presence in a rapidly modernizing Japan. Nonetheless, he acquired notoriety after curing—thanks to his "archaic" techniques and knowledge, relics of a feudal past his contemporaries were eager to forget—the French ambassador Michel Jules Marie Léon Roches, as well as, rumor had it, Prince Yoshihito 嘉仁 (later to be known as Emperor Taishō 大正 天皇). In his 1885 "Notes on the History of Medical Progress in Japan," Willis Norton Whitney reported that Asada, a "physician of the Old, or Chinese School, who follows religiously the teachings of the ancients," and since 1861 personal physician of the shogun, in 1865 was called to the shogunal castle to look at "the French Minister Roches, who had suffered from a disease which had for a number of years baffled all medical skill." Only Asada "succeeded in restoring him to health."[21]

Asada's medical successes were widely publicized at the time, often in open polemic against the *bakufu*'s and, later, the Meiji government's unconditional support of Western medicine. Whitney noted that Asada was like all "*Kuwam-pō-no-isha*, or Chinese educated physicians, as they are called, [who] always dispense their own medicines, which consist for the most part of herbs, and a few mineral substances, as mercury and lime." Throughout his long essay, Whitney severely criticized both the efficacy and the powerful aura of mystery that surrounded these "Chinese educated physicians." He noted, however, with undisguised relief, that "although, among the most conservative of the higher classes, as well as among the lower and ignorant classes, the Chinese physicians are still very popular, the superiority of Western medicine is rapidly becoming apparent to all."[22]

Kanpōyaku physicians were certainly the first to note the increasing support and institutional success of Western medicine—which included substantial financial support from the state. It was to oppose this trend that Asada and other traditional physicians founded the Onchisha 温知社 (Society for the

---

20   Natsume 2001, 420.

21   Whitney 1885, 387.

22   Whitney 1885, 388.

Revival of Wisdom) in 1879, a society for the support of *kanpōyaku*, whose efforts included the foundation of schools in the various prefectures to preserve this medical profession. Most importantly, the Onchisha and its members appealed on various occasions to the government and the Imperial Assembly (Teikoku gikai 帝国議会). The survival of *kanpōyaku* was put in jeopardy in 1879, however, when a system of state examinations for the certification and licensing of physicians trained in state institutions was put into place. Now the medical profession required training in biology, chemistry, anatomy, physics, surgery, diagnostics, pharmacognosy, ophthalmology, etc. This system prohibited de jure and de facto all physicians trained in *kanpōyaku* from practicing medicine, placing them into an uncertain and contradictory legal status whereby it was not clear whether they would be allowed to continue to treat patients or not.

In 1891 a petition signed by 1,984 *kanpōyaku* physicians and 51,050 citizens was sent to the new Imperial Diet to plead for recognition of *kanpōyaku* training and for authorization to practice. The petition was rejected, but it stirred quite a debate among intellectuals and opinion makers over the value of *kanpōyaku* as a diagnostic and treatment technique that soon expanded into a debate over the moral legacy of traditional culture.

It is important to remember that the political and ideological context dramatically changed after the first two decades of the Meiji period. Between 1887 and 1897 the anxious impulse to modernize, Westernize, and repudiate the "feudal" past—the persistent leitmotiv of the Civilization and Enlightenment Movement—had begun to wither away, and in its place a new self-conscious national ideology emerged that was able to accommodate the ideas and practices of instrumental rationality and technological innovation alongside the preservation of a national essence. *Kokutai* 国体—or "national essence," a term imbued with Confucian overtones that was resuscitated from the polemical pamphlets of late Tokugawa political discourse—now became the central keyword of the Imperial Rescript on Education that all schoolchildren had to memorize and religiously recite at the beginning of every school day. This accommodation resulted in a communion of technological advancement and traditional ethics that brought back to life the once anachronistic Tokugawa Confucian legacy.

It is therefore not surprising that the 1891 appeal to the Imperial Diet by *kanpōyaku* physicians was able to mobilize more than fifty thousand supporters among intellectuals, artists, members of the imperial nobility and the high bourgeoisie, and the like. Japan had now achieved a degree of industrial and technological advancement—soon to be proved in the military field against China and Russia for supremacy over East Asia—that no longer necessitated an open disavowal of its "feudal" and "backward" past. The "escape from Asia" (*datsu-A ron* 脱亜論) that inflamed the columns of the newspapers in 1885 had already acquired a different meaning by the 1890s: Japan was ready, on the one hand, to reconcile scientific, industrial, and political modernization with a "national essence" that was now believed to have been slowly precipitated in the Tokugawa ideologico-cultural centrifuge; and it was ready, on the other hand, to lead the awakening of the entirety of East Asia to the necessities of the modern world, a colonial enterprise that the war with China would soon make explicit.[23]

Physicians trained in Western medicine must have felt this change of mood and have believed their authority to be under threat. In 1892 a delegation of modern physicians petitioned the Diet to prohibit once and for all the practice of *kanpōyaku*. The battle for political legitimation continued until 1895, when the Diet established (105 votes against 78) that *kanpōyaku* should not be granted equal status with modern medicine nor should the state legitimate or support *kanpōyaku* as a social service. However, its practice was not outlawed, prohibited, or subjected to control or limitations. It could be privately practiced, and if a certified physician—that is, a physician who had passed the state examination—decided to try a *kanpōyaku* treatment on a patient, then he was legally authorized to do so with the financial support of the state.

At the same time, in the field of *honzōgaku*, Mori Risshi 森立之 (1807–1885), better known by his intellectual pseudonym of Kien 枳園, promoted a revival of old-style *honzōgaku* precisely when the majority of Japanese botanists were translating their traditional knowledge into the language of Western biology. He rejected Li Shizhen's *Bencao gangmu*, which, according to Mori, had abandoned the traditional dialectical conception of medicinal substances as being both therapeutic and poisonous and also had privileged the classification of natural species according to their medicinal effects, that is, had emphasized subjective effects over objects. Mori dedicated his life to the philological recovery of the forms and meanings of the ancient *bencao* tradition. In a quest to reconstruct the lost *Divine Husbandman's Materia Medica* (*Shennong bencao jing*), a text probably compiled around the second and first centuries BCE and now lost), Mori studied Tao Hongjing's 陶弘景 *Bencao jing jizhu* 本草経集注 (*Notes on the Canon of Materia Medica*, ca. 492 CE) along with *Xinxiu bencao* 新修本草 (*Revised Materia Medica*) and Japanese classics of the Heian period like Fukane Sukehito's 深根輔仁 *Honzō wamyō* 本草和名 (*Materia Medica in Japanese*), Minamoto no Shitagō's 源順 *Wamyō ruijushō* 和名類聚抄 (*Thematic Dictionary of Japanese Terms*), and Tanba no Yasuyori's 丹波康頼 *Ishinpō*

---

23   Okakura 1905

医心方 (*Essential Medical Prescriptions*). Mori's initiative was not merely philological nor was it motivated by a vain nostalgia for the past: not only did he
want to restore the tripartite division of "princely," "ministerial," and "adjutant"
drugs to the actual practice of traditional apothecaries and *kanpōyaku* physicians, but he also conceived of his work in open polemic against the modernizing fury of early Meiji Japan, so keen to reject its past.

    Three points of interest can be highlighted in the double story of how in the
early Meiji period *honzōgaku* both lost its name while keeping its cognitive
content and kept its name while disavowing two centuries of Tokugawa research. First, juxtaposed to the intense enthusiasm for modernization and
Westernization in the first two decades of the Meiji period, the lives and works
of Asada Sōhaku and Mori Risshi testified to a resistance to change that has
hardly found mention in the narratives of Japanese modernization. I see their
marginalization in the mainstream historiography of science as a sign of the
ideological ambivalence of the Meiji period itself, caught as it was in an aporia
between modernization/Westernization and the construction of a national
identity. It seems to me that Asada and Mori distinguished themselves by their
estrangement from this dialectic, as they did not substantially contribute to
either one of these two processes and yet in part captured the difficult relation
of Meiji intellectuals with their immediate past. On the one hand, as admirers
and preservers of an idealized past, they stood for what Nietzsche called the
"antiquarian" method of history writing. Nietzsche saw history as being deprived of any inherent meaning in itself and therefore as being constantly as-
cribed meaning and therefore continuously transformed in an incessant
process of interpretation and reinterpretation. The "restricted field of vision"
of antiquarian historians causes them to "assign to the things of the past no
difference in value and proportion which would distinguish things from each
other fairly, but measure things by the proportions of the antiquarian individual or people looking back into the past." Asada and Mori pledged their fidelity to a discipline, a type of knowledge, a technology, and the worldviews
attached to it precisely when they were threatening to vanish. In a sense, Asada
and Mori both lived in the past, as Natsume Sōseki perceptively ironized, as
antiquarians in Nietzsche's sense. Because of their strong commitment to an
orthodox version of their vanishing disciplines, both of them failed to produc-
tively engage with the contemporary intellectual discourse. On the contrary,
they made their estrangement from it a fundamental characteristic of their
own intellectual production and professional activities. As Nietzsche put it,
they were able to preserve life but were not able to generate new life: "When
the sense of a people is hardened like this, when history serves the life of the
past in such a way that it buries further living, especially higher living, when

the historical sense no longer conserves life, but mummifies it, then the tree dies unnaturally, from the top gradually down to the roots, and at last even the roots are generally destroyed. Antiquarian history itself degenerates in that moment when it no longer inspires and fills with enthusiasm the fresh life of the present."[24]

And yet—and this is my second point—the struggle of Asada and Mori did acquire some resonance precisely at the moment when the modernizing impulse of Meiji Japan was giving way to an identitarian discourse centered on the emperor, the national essence, and the construction of a Japanese empire in East Asia. That is, their legal struggle for recognition and legitimation in the 1890s enjoyed a certain visibility because of the change in the ideological strategy of imperial Japan. However, that notoriety—this is my third and last point—ensued independently from what they were defending of *kanpōyaku* and old-style *honzōgaku*. Indeed, I think that neither Asada's nor Mori's antiquarianism had anything to do with identitarian constructions or nationalistic views. Quite the opposite: they defended a typically early modern East Asian cosmopolitanism—a belief in the Sinocentric cultural and intellectual sphere that deeply characterized early modern thought, especially in Japan—that was completely at odds with concepts like national essence (*kokutai*), escape from Asia (*datsu-A ron*), and a darkened, feudal, and backward early modern East Asia that characterized the writings of the thinkers of the Civilization and Enlightenment Movement.

Returning to an original *honzōgaku*, just like preserving the ancient techniques of traditional Chinese medicine (*kanpōyaku*), meant defending and preserving a sense of cultural unity that resisted the language of culturalism and national essentialism of modernity. Antiquarians in a Nietzschean sense, Asada and Mori were indeed surviving relics of a time far past. But it was precisely for that reason that they could be mobilized, in the context of "overcoming modernity," in the early twentieth century, as symbols of a past that was worth protecting in order to recover the possibility of an alternative modernity, a modernity other than, and in opposition to, the West.

References

Barshay, Andrew E. 2004. *The Social Sciences in Modern Japan: The Marxian and Modernist Traditions*. Los Angeles: University of California Press.

Bartholomew, James R. 1989. *The Formation of Science in Japan: Building a Research Tradition*. New Haven, CT: Yale University Press.

---

24   Nietzsche 2010.

Fujita Teiichirō 藤田貞一郎 2003. *Kindai Nihon keizaishi kenkyū no shinshikaku: Kokueki shisō, ichiba, dōgyōkumiai, Robinson hyōryūki* 近代日本経済史研究の新視角：国益思想・市場・同業組合・ロビンソン漂流記 [New approaches to the study of modern Japanese economic history: National prosperity, the market, trade organizations, and *The Adventures of Robinson Crusoe*]. Osaka: Seibundō.

Gluck, Carol 1985. *Japan's Modern Myths: Ideology in the Late Meiji Period*. Princeton, NJ: Princeton University Press.

Gould, Stephen Jay, and Elizabeth S. Vrba 1982. "Exaptation—a Missing Term in the Science of Form," *Paleobiology* 8, 1: 4–15.

Hachisuka Masauji 蜂須賀正氏 2006. *Minami no tanken* 南の探検 [Southern explorations]. Tokyo: Heibonsha.

Kagaku Asahi 科学朝日, ed. 1991. *Tonosama seibutsugaku no keifu* 殿様生物学の系譜 [The genealogy of aristocrats' biology]. Tokyo: Asahi Sensho.

Koerner, Lisbet 2001. *Linnaeus: Nature and Nation*. Cambridge, MA: Harvard University Press.

Kōsaka Masaaki 高坂正顕 1999. *Meiji shisōshi* 明治思想史 [Intellectual history of the Meiji period], edited by Minamoto Ryōen 源了圓. Kyoto: Tōeisha.

Marcon, Federico (forthcoming). *The Knowledge of Nature and the Nature of Knowledge in Early Modern Japan*. Chicago: University of Chicago Press.

Miller, Ian J. 2013. *The Nature of the Beast: Empire and Exhibition at the Tokyo Imperial Zoo*. Los Angeles: University of California Press.

Narita Ryūichi 成田龍一 2002. "Jikan no kindai: Kokumin-kokka no jikan" 時間の近代―国民国家の時間 [The modernity of time: The time of the nation-state], in Komori Yōichi 小森陽一 et al., eds., *Kindai Nihon no bunkashi* 近代日本の文化史 [Cultural history of modern Japan], vol. 3, *Kindai chi no seiritsu* 近代知の成立 [The formation of modern knowledge]. Tokyo: Iwanami shoten, 1–51.

Natsume Sōseki 2001. *I Am a Cat*, translated by Aiko Ito and Graeme Wilson. North Clarendon, VT: Tuttle.

Nietzsche, Friedrich 2010. "On the Use and Abuse of History for Life," translated by Ian Johnston, http://records.viu.ca/~johnstoi/Nietzsche/history.htm (last accessed April 19, 2013).

Nishimura Saburō 西村三郎 1999. *Bunmei no naka no hakubutsugaku: Seiō to Nihon* 文明のなかの博物学: 西欧と日本 [Natural history in civilizations: The West and Japan]. 2 vols. Tokyo: Kinokuniya shoten.

Okakura Kakuzō 1905. *The Awakening of Japan*. New York: Century.

Shimane Kenritsu Daigaku Nishi Amane Kenkyūkai 島根県立大学西周研究会編, ed. 2005. *Nishi Amane to Nihon no kindai* 西周と日本の近代 [Nishi Amane and Japanese modernity]. Tokyo: Perikansha.

Shirai Mitsutarō 白井光太郎 1933. *Jumoku wamyō kō* 樹木和名考 [Reflections on the Japanese names of trees]. Tokyo: Uchida Rōkakuho.

Ueno Masuzō 上野益三 1991. *Hakubutsugakusha retsuden* 博物学者列伝 [Lineages of natural historians]. Tokyo: Yasaka shobō.

Whitney, Willis Norton 1885. "Notes on the History of Medical Progress in Japan," *Transactions of the Asiatic Society of Japan* 12.

Japanese Medical Texts in Chinese on *Kakké* in the Tokugawa and Early Meiji Periods

Angela Ki Che Leung

Introduction

The *kakké* disorder became a focus of medical interest in late Tokugawa and early Meiji Japan when the epidemic was observed in major cities and in the military and even began to affect the imperial household.[1] The main symptoms of the disease included swelling or emaciation, loss of sensation and strength in the legs, sometimes followed by fatal heart failure. It was seen by Japanese elites and authorities as a serious threat to the healthy growth of the rising nation, as the main victims appeared to be able-bodied males, especially young men in the army and navy.[2] The disorder provided a unique occasion for doctors of different medical traditions in Japan to prove the efficacy of their theories and therapeutics. *Kanpō* doctors, versed in Chinese classical medical texts, were the first to observe and comment on the *kakké* phenomenon in modern Japan.

Kakké is now commonly considered to be the equivalent of beriberi, which is defined in biomedicine as "a nutritional disorder due to deficiency of vitamin B1 (thiamine) ... widespread in rice-eating communities in which the diet is based on polished rice, from which the thiamine-rich seed coat has been removed." The symptoms, including the weakness of the legs and the ultimately fatal heart condition, are the result of nervous degeneration caused by the

---

*   This paper is based on research funded by the Research Grant Council of the Hong Kong government for my project "Medical Culture in the Canton-Hong Kong Region in the Long Nineteenth Century" (Project No. HKU 446909H, 2009–2012).

1   *Kakké* moved to the center of attention during the Seinan civil war of 1877. Many of the troops fell sick with this disease, with a rate of affliction in the army of 11 percent in 1876, climbing to 14 percent in 1877 and 38 percent in 1878. Beginning in April 1876, the Japanese empress suffered from this disease; in 1877 the emperor's sister died from it. See Oberlander 2005, 15.

2   See Bay 2006.

deficiency of thiamine.[3] This interpretation of *kakké* was established and widely accepted only in the interwar period of the twentieth century, with the Nobel Prize in Medicine granted to the British chemist F. G. Hopkins and the Dutch physician C. Eijkman for their work leading to the discovery of vitamins. Eijkman's contribution was specifically the successful framing of beriberi as a deficiency disease caused by the exclusive consumption of polished white rice. The disease was basically unknown to European scientists before Eijkman published the findings of his experiments with chickens fed on white rice in the Dutch East Indies in the last decades of the nineteenth century.

Kakké 脚氣 is the Japanese pronunciation of the same Chinese word for an ailment described in early Chinese medical classics. The Chinese term, *jiaoqi* 脚氣, literally meaning "leg-*qi*," highlighted the effects on the legs, along with *qi*, perverse "Wind," as the supposed cause of the disease. Both the Chinese and Japanese terms are represented by the same Chinese characters. The term *jiaoqi* appeared in early Chinese medical classics not later than the fourth century and was discussed as a major disease category in medical texts thereafter, with a high point from the seventh to the early twelfth centuries.[4] Recent research cautions against the simplistic translation of *jiaoqi* in classical Chinese medical texts, thus also of *kakké*, as the beriberi defined by modern biomedicine.[5] The history of *jiaoqi/kakké* has been made opaque and impenetrable because malnutrition, a modern biomedical construct of the first decades of the twentieth century,[6] increasingly has reduced the etiological complexity of beriberi to single, context-free biochemical factors.[7] The deficiency explanation of beriberi, moreover, has left many features of modern *jiaoqi/kakké* (and even of beriberi) unexplained.[8] In this paper I will attempt to partially restore

---

3   *The Bantam Medical Dictionary* 2000, 52.

4   See Smith 2008; Ryō 1936, 11–32.

5   Smith 2008; Liao 2001, 2011.

6   Worboys 1988; Arnold 1994; Kamminga and Cunningham 1995.

7   For example, in his 1961 book, Robert Williams promotes the enrichment of rice and bread with thiamine as a straightforward solution to eradicating beriberi; for a critique of such a position, see Scrinis 2008.

8   Features that remained unexplained included the seasonal factor (the epidemics were more acute in warm months) and gender differences (most patients were men). The white-rice theory also could not explain the prevalence of beriberi in nineteenth-century southern China, where most Chinese of the time could not afford expensive polished white rice, and their diet was rarely exclusively limited to rice. Questions on such issues raised in international forums such as the congresses of the Far Eastern Association of Tropical Medicine in the early twentieth century were never fully answered. See also Liao 2001.

the social and cultural context in which *kanpō* doctors observed and understood the *kakké* epidemic in modern Japan. I will do this by surveying explanations of the disorder in *kanpō* medical texts of the eighteenth and early nineteenth centuries prior to the domination of biomedicine in Japanese public health around the turn of the century.

The *kakké* epidemic observed in the late Tokugawa period was understood, analyzed, and debated with traditional *kanpō* categories. In the 1853 compilation by Taki Motokata 多紀元堅 (also known as Tanba Genken 丹波元堅, 1795–1857), *kakké* was given a comprehensive description based on old Chinese and *kanpō* texts: as a disease caused by the intrusion of the Wind toxin (*fūdoku* 風毒),[9] *kakké* caused sluggishness in the legs, head, neck, or shoulder. Taki also described the "wet" and "dry" types of *kakké*, the former characterized by swollenness, the latter by emaciation and dryness of the skin and numbness in the lower abdomen. In keeping with classical Chinese explanations of the ailment, the toxin was said to enter the patient's body by penetrating the lower limbs and moving up. When it reached the Heart, the patient would die.[10] The death caused by the toxin's finally attacking the Heart (*shōshin* 衝心) was the key feature of the clinical pattern of *kakké*, justifying the great public attention paid to the growing epidemic.

At the beginning of the eighteenth century, Japanese doctors began to notice an increase in the incidence of *kakké*, and between the 1710s and 1861, at least twenty-eight *kanpō* monographs on *kakké* were published.[11] Given that single-disease medical texts were rare in both classical Chinese and Japanese traditions, this figure is revealing. In his *On Recipes to Treat* Kakké (*Kakké hōron* 脚氣方論, 1748), Matsui Zaian 松井材庵 (also known as Matsui Etsushū 松井閱眾 and Matsui Shūsuke 松井眾甫) claimed that the prevalence of *kakké* had been noticeable for some thirty years, affecting the nobility as well as the common people, many of whom died of the disease.[12] Calling the ailment *eyami* 瘟, Matsui appeared to consider the *kakké* of the early eighteenth century a contagious epidemic comparable to those that had been caused by the warm factor and had been prevalent in China since the mid-seventeenth

---

9   "Wind toxin" (*fengdu* 風毒 in Chinese) was already described as the cause of *jiaoqi* in *Handy Recipes for Urgent Situations* (*Zhou houbeiji fang* 肘後備急方), one of the earliest Chinese medical classics, by Ge Hong 葛洪 (283–343), that mentioned the ailment. Both Sun Simiao 孫思邈 (ca. 581–682) and Chao Yuanfang 巢元方 (active early seventh century) used the term to explain *jiaoqi* in their medical writings.

10   Taki (1853) 1983, 124–126.

11   Liao 2001, 125–126, quoting Fujii Naohisa 藤井尚久, *The History of Our Nation's Diseases* (*Honpō shippei shi*《本邦疾病史》).

12   Matsui 1766.

century.[13] *Kakké* was managed as a particular public health threat only in the late nineteenth century when Nakano Yasuaki 淺田宗伯 (1813–1894), a leading *kanpō* doctor, set up the first *kanpō* hospital, the Hakusai byōin 博濟病院 (Hospital for General Relief), in 1878 to treat *kakké* patients. This hospital claimed a low mortality rate of 2 percent among these patients, competing favorably with the state *kakké* hospital that used both *Kanpō* and biomedicine. For *kanpō* doctors of this period, the *kakké* epidemic was an exceptional opportunity to redress the authority of *kanpō* medicine, now being seriously challenged by biomedical doctors.[14]

The discussions on the *kakké* epidemic by *kanpō* doctors were based essentially on Chinese medical classics produced in the medieval period from the Sui to the Song dynasties, roughly from the seventh to twelfth centuries, when *jiaoqi* was a much-discussed ailment.[15] Late imperial medical experts, especially those after the fourteenth century, seem to have lost interest in studying the disease. A compilation of therapeutic recipes attributed to a high Qing scholar-official from Guangdong, He Mengyao 何夢瑤 (1693–1764), remained in manuscript form until 1918 and did not offer any new explanations on the ailment.[16] A "revival" of interest in the disease only came about in the late nineteenth and early twentieth centuries, when He's manuscript was finally published in Canton. A doctor from Guangdong, having worked in a Hong Kong charitable hospital, published a major new work in 1887 (see below). The relative lack of interest in *jiaoqi* in the eighteenth and earlier part of the nineteenth centuries in China contrasts intriguingly with the great importance attached to *kakké* by *kanpō* doctors and the Japanese authorities of the same period, who produced a much richer literature on the disease, with new interpretations of classical theories. This general Chinese disregard for the *jiaoqi* disorder was probably one main reason why the American doctor Duane Simmons, of the China Imperial Maritime Customs, believed, in the 1880s, that the

---

13   On epidemiology in late imperial China, see Hanson 2011, esp. chap. 1, on "warm diseases."

14   Nakano and Asada (1879) 1993, preface, 1; postface, 46; "On the Hospital for General Relief," 47–48; Pan and Fan 1994, 209.

15   There was even a monograph on the ailment published in the late eleventh century by Dong Ji 董汲 that is no longer extant but was partially retrieved from fragments during the early Ming. Parts of Dong Ji's *Essentials of Jiaoqi Therapeutics* (*Jiaoqi zhifa zongyao* 腳氣治法總要), in two *juan*, are available in the early Ming encyclopedia *Yongle dadian* and reprinted in the 1924 Sansan Medical Collection (*Sansan yishu*) edited by Qiu Qingyuan.

16   He 1918.

beriberi/*kakké* then endemic in the Dutch East Indies and Japan did not exist in China.[17]

This essay will look at the discussions on *kakké* in *kanpō* texts of the late Tokugawa and early Meiji period (ca. 1748–1883) that were influential not only in Japan but also read and even published in China.[18] I will analyze the nature and etiological construction of the ailment by *kanpō* authors, which were first based on traditional Chinese concepts of *jiaoqi* and later on additional, new anatomical knowledge introduced by Western experts, and I will show how such explanations made sense of the social and cultural problems generated by the urban lifestyle emerging in Japan. I will then briefly compare these explanations with late Qing Chinese medical texts on *jiaoqi* to highlight the particularities of the Japanese context of the modern *kakké* epidemic. I will try to show why, in the complex and rapidly changing political, social, and cultural environment of modern Asia where the *kakké/jiaoqi* epidemics were developing, it was difficult for doctors and patients in Japan and China to understand and accept a biochemical deficiency theory focusing on polished white rice as the sole cause.

Japanese *Kakké*: An Elusive and Changing Disease

One salient feature running through most of the *kanpō* texts in the period under study was the claim that the *kakké* observed in Japan then was the same as the *jiaoqi* disorder described in Chinese Tang and Song medical classics. This justified the authors' use of these classics as basic references to check against popular recipes alleged to be effective therapeutics. *Kanpō* doctors often stressed the "authenticity" of knowledge on *kakké* as compared with the adulterated information on diseases bearing the same name described in the late imperial period. In one of the earlier texts, Minamoto Yasunori's 源養德 *Recipes on* Kakké (*Kakké ruihō* 腳氣類方, 1763), the author wrote in the preface that "the discussion on *kakké* during the Tang/Song period is correct and standard; Yuan/Ming doctors' discussions are mostly irrelevant, and one does not take them seriously. The book *Recipes Worth a Thousand Gold Pieces*[19] [by Sun Simiao 孫思邈, 581–682] is the most essential and standard. As for the book by

17   Simmons 1880, 40.

18   All the texts cited in this essay are kept in major medical libraries in China and recorded in their catalogs.

19   *Beiji qianjin yaofang* 備急千金要方 (ca. 650–659).

Wang Tao 王燾 [670–755],[20] though thorough, it is too dense and thick, whereas the two collections of recipes [of the Song dynasty], *Shenghui* 聖惠 and
Shengji 聖濟,[21] do synthesize various theories, with tested, fine recipes."[22]
With minor differences, *kanpō* doctors writing on *kakké* agreed on these classical texts as the core of the corpus for the study of the disease.

Taki Motokata, author of *Broad Essentials of Various Diseases* (*Zatsubyō kōyō*
雜病廣要, 1853), in keeping with Minamoto Yasunori's analyses of *kakké*, was
more specific. He reiterated the conviction that the *jiaoqi* described in Tang
texts was the same as Japanese *kakké*, whereas the *jiaoqi* discussed after the
Song was often confused with ordinary numbness and pain of the legs, very
different from the *kakké* that would develop into fatal heart attacks (*shōshin*).
The two Song imperial recipe collections cited by Minamoto Yasunori also
served as basic references for *kanpō* authors on *kakké* therapeutics. In 1812, for
example, Okamoto Shōan 岡本昌庵 published a monograph of recipes based
on the *Recipes of the Imperial Grace during the Great Peace* (*Taiping shenghui*
fang 太平聖惠方, 992).[23] An 1811 book by Maruyama Genshō 丸山元璋, however, shows that for some Tokugawa *kanpō* doctors of the early nineteenth century, the importance of *kakké* was still uncertain. He called the disease "a minor
ailment" (*shōshitsu* 小疾), not worthy of the attention of great doctors, even
though he already observed a growing number of patients falling sick between
summer and autumn. Based also on Sun Simiao's classic, Maruyama's work reflected divided opinion on the seriousness of the epidemic in Japan even in the
early nineteenth century despite the visible increase in prevalence, in contrast
to the unquestionable consensus on its identification with *jiaoqi* as discussed
in Chinese medieval classics.[24]

Even though *kanpō* doctors took Chinese medieval medical classics as the
ultimate authority on the *kakké* problem, they also emphasized the intangible
character of the epidemic observed during their time. A second consensus
among *kanpō* authors on *kakké* was that, despite the claimed affinity of the
modern Japanese epidemic with early medieval Chinese *jiaoqi*, *kakké* was not
exactly the same as *jiaoqi*, especially in terms of etiology, but was a "transformed" version of the old disease. In the late eighteenth century Minamoto

---

20   *Medical Secrets from the Royal Library* (*Waitai miyao fang* 外臺秘要, ca. 752).

21   By *Shenghui* 聖惠 he is referring to *Recipes of the Imperial Grace during the Great Peace*
     (*Taiping sheng hui fang* 太平聖惠方, 992). *Shengji* 聖濟 refers to *General Record of Impe-*
     rial Charity (*Shengji zonglu* 聖濟總錄, eleventh century).

22   Minamoto (1763) 1899, 4a.

23   Okamoto 1812.

24   Maruyama 1811, 1a.

had already characterized *kakké* as mutable in time and place: *kakké* in medieval times was not the same as that in the present, and that occurring in the north was different from that in the south.[25] Similarly, Taki Motokata later stressed the mutable character of *kakké* by highlighting the possibility that, just as modern *kakké* was similar to Tang and Song *jiaoqi* and different from the *jiaoqi* of the Yuan and Ming periods, *kakké* in the future might very well differ from the disorder they observed in their time, so that taking measures that corresponded to the situation at the time was key to the successful treatment of the epidemic.[26] Imamura Ryō 今村亮 (also known as Imamura Ryōan 今村了奄, 1841–1890), court physician of the Tokugawa family and an authority on *kakké*, wrote in his seminal book on the disease published in 1861, *Essentials on* Kakké (*Kakké kōyō* 腳氣鉤要), that experience suggested to him that ancient *kakké* might not be the same as the modern disease, which inspired him to modify old recipes to treat the modern.[27] As someone who lived in a rapidly changing era, he understandably stressed the mutability of all diseases: "All diseases under heaven are subject to change according to time and place. The changes are also infinite." Therapeutics, therefore, had to be very flexible.[28]

The mutability of *kakké* was further elaborated by Nakano Yasuaki 岡田昌春 and Asada Sōhaku 淺田惟常 (director of the Hospital for General Relief in 1878), who published the *General Treatise on* Kakké (*Kakké gairon* 腳氣概論) in 1879, where they developed the idea that *kakké* was an elusive disorder that changed with time and place. The reason for their compiling the book was that, despite the mentions of the disease in old Tang and Song classics and in old *kanpō* texts such as *Ishinpō* 醫心方 (tenth century) and *Man'anpō* 萬安方 (fourteenth century), the effectiveness of recipes and therapeutics depended on locality and customs, time and circumstances. The authors quoted old *kanpō* classics to prove that "in our country, the disease had existed for a thousand years." However, "in later times, when the four seas were in great turmoil with incessant warfare, we rarely heard of the disease again. In recent years, [this illness] has reemerged. The clinical patterns are similar to those described in Jin and Tang medical classics. The analyses are also similar. This is due to changing times and customs. We are in a different era."[29] The authors seemed to imply here that *kakké* was a disease of prosperity and peace. *Kakké* reappeared in peaceful and affluent Meiji Japan, real *jiaoqi* was endemic in

---

25   Minamoto (1763) 1899, 10a.
26   Taki (1853) 1983, 120.
27   Imamura 1861, *juan* 1, *hanrei* 凡例 (explanatory notes), 1a.
28   Imamura 1861, *juan* 1, 15b.
29   Nakano and Asada (1879) 1993, 5.

prosperous Tang China, and the disorder bearing the same name was likely to have been confused with other diseases in turbulent late imperial China. They went on to assert, under the section heading "On the Differences in Clinical Patterns between Old and Modern *Kakké* in This Nation," that modern *kakké* characterized by the fatal heart attack, as described in Han and Tang classics, was first observed in Japan only in the Hōreki 寶曆 era (1751–1764). Moreover, the *kakké* in modern Japan was also characterized by its prevalence in the warmer season, from summer to autumn, and affected mostly young and able-bodied males, features that were not analyzed in medieval Chinese classics on *jiaoqi*.[30]

Imamura Ryō, in his later syncretic work on the disease, *New Treatise on Kakké* (*Kakké shinron* 腳氣新論, 1878), again summarized his views on the elusive nature of disease and the specificity of modern epidemics prevalent in urbanized and prosperous Meiji Japan: "Diseases are complex; their changes are multiple. There are modern diseases that did not exist in the past, such as cholera. And there are modern diseases that became more prominent than in the past, such as *kakké*."[31] For Imamura and other *kanpō* doctors of the mid-nineteenth century, cholera and *kakké* marked Japan's modernity in significant ways: devastating mostly densely populated urban hubs and victimizing well-off and able-bodied young men in great numbers, the diseases seemed to be the by-products of development and prosperity. This idea was behind most of the discussions on the etiology of *kakké* by *kanpō* doctors.

The perception of a mutable *kakké* was articulated more and more clearly in major *kanpō* texts, a feature that was totally absent in contemporary Chinese medical texts. *Kanpō* writers since the early eighteenth century were aware that they were living in a rapidly changing time and experiencing "new" diseases with particular transmission patterns corresponding to new social contexts and mores. Such diseases were seen as necessary evils of an increasingly affluent, rapidly transforming, and urbanizing nation.

Causes of *Kakké*: Intangible Wind and Damp Toxins

Most *kanpō* writers maintained that the Wind toxin (*fūdoku* 風毒) was the main cause of *kakké*. The Chinese equivalent, *fengdu*, as in the title of the *jiaoqi* chapter in Sun Simiao's classic, was used as the collective term to include all external pathogens (Cold, Heat, Wind, Dampness) emerging from the ground. As one's legs were in constant and direct contact with the ground, they were

---

30   Nakano and Asada (1879) 1993, 5–6.

31   Imamura 1878, preface, 2a.

the first part of the body to be affected by the toxin, thus the term leg-*qi*. The toxin would then move up the body and when it reached and attacked the Heart, the patient would die.[32] This fatal development of *jiaoqi*, according to *kanpō* experts, distinguished real *jiaoqi*, or *kakké*, from other leg and foot ailments described in post-Song medical texts. Based on this classical definition of *fengdu*, *kanpō* experts further revised and elaborated the notion to accommodate their idea of an elusive *kakké*. While both Tachibana Genshu 橘元周 (also called Katakura Kakuryō 片倉鶴陵, 1751–1822), in his 1787 monograph on *kakké*,[33] and Taki Motokata adhered to Sun's explanations, considering the toxin to be the usual external pathogens, Imamura Ryō, in an effort to distinguish Japanese *kakké* from Chinese *jiaoqi*, constructed the concept of "Damp toxin" (*suidoku* 水毒), a toxin different from the usual external pathogens, emerging from the ground only in summer and autumn.[34] In his later synthesis of *kakké*, he provided a totally different interpretation of *fūdoku*: the disease was attributed to "Wind," or *ki*, not so much because of the importance of the implied external pathogens, but because the two terms defined the disease's elusive and mutative character. To him, the toxin that caused *kakké* was not just any external pathogen under the umbrella of *fūdoku* but a compressed severe toxin (*utsudoku* 欝毒) buried deep underground,[35] an idea reminiscent of the *zaqi* 雜氣 (malignant *qi*) concept that the late Ming doctor Wu Youxing 吳有性 used to explain the series of contemporary epidemics in Jiangnan.[36]

The revised etiology of *kakké* as having roots in but different from that of the medieval Chinese *jiaoqi* corresponded to the doctors' understanding of the changing environment of a unique, modernizing, and urbanizing Japan. *kanpō* doctors seemed to be most impressed by the main victims of the disorder: formerly healthy and often well-off urban men. In his 1787 monograph on *kakké*, Tachibana Genshu had already noted that these main victims dwelled in luxury mansions and enjoyed a rich diet and a leisurely life. To explain this new and unusual phenomenon, however, he relied on the Chinese medical concept of fetal toxin (*taidoku, taidu* 胎毒), a poison introduced into the fetus during intercourse between sexual partners with excessive carnal passion.[37] What was implied here was obviously a perceived hedonistic lifestyle in urban Japan that

---

32   Sun (1307) 1955, *juan* 7, "Fengdu jiaoqi," 138–140.
33   Tachibana 1787, preface, 1b.
34   Imamura 1861, *juan* 2, 1a.
35   Imamura 1878, 1b–2b.
36   For a recent discussion on Wu Youxing and his impact, see Hanson 2011, chap. 5.
37   The concept was a relatively late invention, appearing in the late Song and especially in the Yuan period, and was most often used to explain childhood diseases such as smallpox. See Chang 2000.

raised the level of fetal toxin in the body. Tachibana warned that excessive sex would unnecessarily boost the Blood and *ki* of the body, further intensifying this innate fetal toxin and making the body extremely receptive to external pathogens. For him fetal toxin was also the cause of other difficult illnesses of the leisurely class such as heat exhaustion, madness, and shoulder pain. The term "Wind toxin" (*fūdoku*), for him, suggested not ordinary external pathogens as stated by Sun Simiao but the extraordinary swiftness of the onslaught of *kakké* on the young and strong, like "galloping horses." The explanation for why fewer women got the disease was that menstruation regularly ridded the fetal toxin from their bodies.[38]

Later *kanpō* doctors of the mid- and late nineteenth century, however, did not take up the fetal toxin explanation but provided new interpretations of the etiological principles of Tang classics. Taki, for example, in his 1853 text, elaborated on the external and internal causes developed by Song and Yuan doctors to explain why the well-to-do were more vulnerable. As the ailment was externally caused by dampness in the ground, Taki claimed that leisurely and immobile people, such as hardworking scholars who remained motionless for a long time on wet ground, and people who engaged in excessive sexual activities without covering their legs properly were the most vulnerable victims; whereas those who enjoyed rich foods and consumed excessive quantities of alcohol and dairy products would contract the disease internally because the intake of such hot and damp foods would provoke stagnation in the lower Burner (abdomen) and consequently swelling in the legs.[39] Two decades later, Imamura further elaborated on a moralizing etiological discourse that tried to make sense of Japan's modernization and urbanization. In his 1878 text, he noted the prevalence of the epidemic especially in metropolitan centers such as Edo, Kyoto, and Naniwa (Osaka). Agreeing with earlier doctors that the epidemic was the result of the hedonistic and decadent lifestyle of wealthy urbanites, he highlighted the internal cause to explain why the wealthy fell ill: excessive food and sex depleted the body of its primordial *ki* (*genki* 元氣), making it vulnerable to external pathogens.[40] Despite *kanpō* doctors' claim that their knowledge of *kakké* was based essentially on Tang and Song classics, Imamura's interpretation shows that they also inherited from Jin and Yuan doctors the reconstructed "internal" causes of diseases, implying the greater personal and moral responsibility of the patient for contracting the disease.[41]

---

38   Tachibana 1787, 1b–2b, 3b–4a. The menstruation theory was also used by late imperial Chinese doctors to explain why there were fewer female victims of leprosy.

39   Taki (1853) 1983, 121–122.

40   Imamura 1878, 3a–b.

41   See Liang 2002, 177–179.

Nakano and Asada explicitly quoted Li Gao 李杲 1180/81–1251/52, one of the four great Jin/Yuan doctors, in their etiological discussion: people who were accustomed to a rich diet of dairy products and alcohol (thus, northerners) would introduce excessive dampness into the body, causing *kakké*.[42] Imamura pushed the "internal" cause argument further to highlight the moral aspect of *kakké* etiology. In modern Japan, he said, urban men in their prime indulging in excessive sex and a luxurious lifestyle were the most vulnerable to the disease, whereas women, children, and the elderly (those excluded from such a lifestyle) were rarely affected. He even provided some crude figures to prove his point: urban, well-to-do males made up 80–90 percent of *kakké* patients.[43]

It was also Imamura who spelled out most clearly, in his 1878 work, why *kakké* was a disease of "modernity." In this book, he reinterpreted the notion of Wind toxin (the *fūdoku* of Sun Simiao) by evoking a new element, toxic air buried beneath urban ground: "wherever the land is lowly and damp, with dense populations and overwhelming human activities, where people do not even have enough space to stand on, the *ki* of the ground, not being able to dissipate freely, will cause this disease. Why then does it emerge only in the spring and summer? It is because [during this season] the *ki* of the ground is on the rise, and as it gets blocked [by human masses and activities on the ground], the obstructed steaming process produces a toxic *ki*."[44] Here, the hedonistic lifestyle of urbanites becomes a secondary cause of *kakké*. Imamura's association of the toxic *ki* with coastal, low-lying, crowded urban settings showed his sensitivity to the changing, modern Japanese context of a "mutable" disease bearing an old name, though the introduction of the miasma in Japan in the early nineteenth century by Dutch doctors probably helped to inspire this reinterpretation.[45]

---

42 Nakano and Asada (1879) 1993, 6. For Li Gao, the main difference was between northern and southern diet and customs. The food and drink of northerners were so rich that there could be accumulation of fluid and heat internally that would slowly descend to the lower limbs, causing *jiaoqi*, whereas southerners would contract the same disease by external pathogens, mainly by the intrusion of external dampness and heat into their bodies.

43 Imamura 1878, 3b–4a. Imamura also stressed that roughly half of the victims (50–60 percent) were attacked by *kakké* while suffering from other diseases: complications from other diseases such as Wind Attack by Cold Damage, fever, distension of the abdomen, diarrhea, lower-abdomen pain with Mold toxin, and postnatal complications for women patients. See Imamura 1861, *juan* 1, 1b.

44 Imamura 1878, 3a.

45 Anthonius F. Baudouin (1822–1885) was one such Dutch doctor. Satomi Giichiro considered miasma a kind of "mold" (*baishu*), a concept close to Imamura's.

Clinical Patterns

Compared with the changing concepts of the origin and causes of *kakké*, the clinical patterns of the disorder remained relatively stable or unchanged. All *kanpō* authors referred to Sun Simiao's classic on the main patterns: "At the beginning, the legs are weak and cannot move easily. Or before anything else, the head, neck, arms, and shoulder suffer, or the heart and abdomen feel sluggish. One may have nausea seeing food and hate the smell of food. There is perhaps diarrhea or constipation and difficulty in urination, unusual throbbing of the heart, the fear of light, or lethargy, forgetfulness, delirium, fever, and headache, coldness and cramping of the body, the ankles may become swollen, legs may feel numb ... numbness also of the lower abdomen." The final and fatal phase of *jiaoqi* was sudden death caused by the malignant *qi* (*shōshin*) attacking the Heart. In his 1861 text, Imamura called for great attentiveness to the slightest symptoms, as they were difficult to detect, especially changes in breathing and urination. Shortness of breath and reddish urine reflected a serious accumulation of internal toxin, whereas unprovoked perspiration and vomiting might indicate the imminence of sudden death.[46]

Using new Western anatomical concepts, Imamura later revised his descriptions of *kakké*. After having worked with biomedical doctors in the state *kakké* hospital, he put aside the Damp-toxin idea and elaborated on the internal "blockage" narrative using Western anatomical categories in his *New Treatise on* Kakké of 1878:[47] for him, the toxin emerging from the ground entered the body first through the legs and then penetrated into liquid blood in blood vessels (i.e., not Blood in the traditional Blood-*ki* duo but the physical, liquid blood of Western anatomy). He also used new anatomical concepts to describe the process of toxin penetration: it first penetrated the skin, then the nerves, the muscles, and, finally and fatally, the viscera. When the toxin entered the heart and the lung via nerve number five, he explained, the case became critical and often terminal. For him, this explained why the fundamental clinical patterns of *kakké* consisted of urinary and breathing abnormalities. The former was a manifestation of the toxin "blocking blood vessels," while the latter was the symptom of the toxin entering the brain and consequently interfering with

---

46   Imamura 1861, *juan* 1, 2a–3a.

47   Imamura 1878, 6b–7b. By this time Imamura, together with Toda Choan 遠田澄庵, had been in contact with his biomedical colleagues, including Kobayashi Tan 小林恒 (1847–1894), Sasaki Toyo 佐佐木東洋 (1838–1918), Ikeda Kensai 池田謙齋 (1841–1918), and Miyake Hiizu 三宅秀 (1848–1938). All of them worked together at the national *kakké* hospital, the Hospital for General Relief, founded by Nagayo Sensai 長與專齋 (1838–1902). See Oberlander 2005, 16–17.

the normal contraction of the heart, leading to lung dysfunction, as the heart and the lungs were interdependent. The fatal and final *shōshin* symptom of *kakké* was, therefore, not "heart attack" but "suffocation" as a result of lung failure.[48] New Western anatomical knowledge, instead of being an effective tool for unseating the explanations and analyses in the *kanpō* classics, provided Imamura, on the contrary, with a new and useful body map with which to consolidate, using a new, modernized vocabulary, the old description of the disease's clinical pattern as established in the classics.

Therapeutics

Kanpō doctors reiterated the difficulty of treating *kakké* because of the deadliness of the toxin.[49] All repeated Sun Simiao's guiding principle that the art of the cure was in maintaining the delicate balance between purging and replenishment, as the illness was caused by both the internal accumulation of toxic matters, blocking the circulation of *ki*, and the depletion of primordial *ki*. Imamura Ryō elaborated on the principle of the dual treatment of "replenish and purge" (*hosha* 補瀉). As "purging accelerated death, and replenishment shortened life," the art was to achieve the perfect balance in the implementation of the two methods. Imamura reminded readers that Chinese medieval classics prioritized purging over replenishment, as most patients died of severe internal stagnation of the toxic *ki*, while purgatives rarely killed.[50] *Kanpō* doctors nonetheless had varied views on the method for purging and regulating *ki*. Earlier doctors such as Minamoto Yasunori, in keeping with the conviction that the disease had been best understood by Sun Simiao, stressed the importance of acupuncture as an essential treatment, especially at the beginning of illness when the patient felt weakness in the legs.[51] He recommended supplementing acupuncture with life-nurturing exercise, *dōin* 導引.[52] Bathing of the legs and applying hot pads to the feet were considered harmful and were generally prohibited.[53]

---

48   Imamura 1878, 7a–b. Imamura also applied the anatomical notions of nerves and muscles in his "new" explanation of *kakké*. Since he stressed the importance of abnormal urination as a major feature of the clinical pattern, he recommended that patients have a urine test.

49   Imamura 1878, postface.

50   Imamura 1861, *juan* 1, 8b–9b.

51   Sun (1307) 1955, 140.

52   Minamoto (1763) 1899, *hanrei* 凡例, *furoku* 附錄 (appendix), 6a–10b.

53   Nakano and Asada (1879) 1993, *hanrei*, 2.

Most *kanpō* doctors in the nineteenth century, however, simply summarized the acupunctural principles of Sun Simiao and Wang Tao without further comment, but they elaborated greatly on drug therapy, as did mainstream doctors in late imperial China. Imamura considered acupuncture "not a method to deal with [the disease's] fundamental causes" but still useful for the removal of obstruction.[54] He stressed the superiority of *kanpō* herbal formulas in treating the Japanese body, especially when compared with Western therapeutics, which he considered to be too abrasive. *kanpō* recipes, he explained, offered patients with made-to-order, composite herbal prescriptions that could target every single symptom of the complicated *kakké* clinical pattern like a well-organized regiment.[55] Here he highlighted the adaptability of therapeutics for patients of different localities and customs. More important still, following the moralizing etiology of *kakké*, *kanpō* doctors prescribed strict bodily discipline as a preventive measure and as a cure, strongly advising against rich diets and overindulgence in sex and alcohol. Imamura recommended unsalted and simple foods, regulated sex, and the control of extreme emotions. Taki Motokata basically advised against alcohol and all meats and vegetables with strong tastes and recommended certain cereals, milk, and chestnuts. While restraining from excessive sex, one must also have moderate exercise, especially walking. Idleness and lying in bed all the time were considered a dangerous lifestyle.[56]

Despite *kanpō* doctors' receptiveness to Western miasmatic theory, most seemed skeptical of Western doctors' advice to remove patients from the place where they had contracted the disease (*tenchi* 轉地, "to change location"). The American doctor Duane Simmons, working in Yokohama in the late nineteenth century, was a typical supporter of such a treatment. He suggested in 1880, "An early removal of the patient beyond the influence of the poison is the best means of treatment," given "no drug has been discovered possessing specific properties in this disease."[57] This method had apparently become one of the most common practices used by Western doctors to treat *kakké* patients in Japan as well as in other parts of colonized Asia,[58] but it was considered with great skepticism by *kanpō* doctors. Tōyama Chinkichi 遠山椿吉 pointed out in 1913 that moving patients to the seaside and low ground, much recom-

---

54   Imamura 1861, *juan* 2, 33a.

55   Imamura 1878, 8a.

56   Imamura 1861, *juan* 1, 2b–3a and the section on "food restrictions" (9b–10a). Nakano and
         Asada ([1879] 1993, *hanrei*, 2) advised patients to strictly respect taboos and life-nurturing
         principles; see also Taki (1853) 1983, 143–144.

57   Simmons 1880, 75–76.

58   The immediate removal of patients from the place where they contracted beriberi was
         also common practice in colonies such as Hong Kong and the Malay states.

mended by Western doctors, would not do any good but would only accelerate the fatal *shōshin* because these places were too damp. He suggested moving patients to high and dry ground if relocation was done at all.[59] The fear of cold damp *ki* and of the toxin buried under city ground, main causes of the disease in classical Chinese and *kanpō* medicine, was behind reservations about moving patients from the place of disease contraction.

Kakké as a Distinct Disease of the Modern Japanese Nation

Kanpō specialists on *kakké* of the eighteenth and nineteenth centuries persistently saw the disease as specific to Japan at that time, a Japan that was characterized by new wealth and accompanying moral corruption. Shortly before the Meiji era, *kanpō* doctors were already seeing *kakké* as a unique, new "old" disease in Japan. Asada Sōhaku, in the postface adorning Imamura's 1861 text, explained the particularity of Japanese *kakké*: "the name [of the ailment] is the same throughout the ages, yet the ailment itself is different; the Japanese and the Chinese descriptions of the clinical patterns are the same and yet the causes are different."[60] Such a perception influenced even some nineteenth-century Western medical specialists who were beginning to take closer looks at what they considered a new disease unknown in the West. In Simmons's 1880 report on the disease for the China Imperial Maritime Customs, he regretted that the name *kakké* was used by all the foreign physicians observing the disease in Japan, "as it is likely to lead to confusion by implying that it is a distinct malady; whereas its identity with beriberi has never been really disputed by anyone but Dr Hoffman."[61]

Actually, not only Hoffman but also the Dutch doctor Pompe van Meerdevort (1829–1908), teacher of Sasaki Toyo (1838–1918) of the government *kakké* hospital, described the Japanese "variation" of beriberi.[62] Simmons himself was contradictory about the specificity of the Japanese *kakké* in relation to beriberi: he conceded that Western doctors, who first observed beriberi in India, understood the disease as being provoked by anemia or malaria and thus treated patients with iron supplements and quinine, killing many Japanese *kakké* patients in the process. He admitted that Japanese doctors' treatment by

---

59   Tōyama 1913, 61.
60   Imamura 1861, postface.
61   Simmons 1880, 39. According to Simmons, the said Dr. Hoffman was misled by his ignorance of Indian beriberi. Simmons believed that beriberi was the same as *kakké*.
62   Oberlander 2005, 18.

"rapid depletion and evacuation of the enormous collections of serous fluid," on the contrary, saved a lot of lives.[63] *Kanpō* etiology and therapeutics of *kakké* obviously enjoyed considerable success and influence in Japan in the late nineteenth century, drawing attention even from foreign biomedical doctors and contributing to the perception of *kakké* as a distinctly Japanese disease.

The claim that *kakké* was a "national" disease of modern Japan can also be appreciated in the sense that the Japanese were among the first to notice the emergence of a new epidemic that needed to be studied seriously. The outbreak of beriberi in the Dutch East Indies was observed and researched by Western biomedical experts only in the last decades of the nineteenth century.[64] The modern *jiaoqi* epidemic in China, on the other hand, remained largely obscure until the early twentieth century. As late as 1905, the government bacteriologist in Hong Kong, like Simmons two decades earlier, reported, "There is no strong proof that the disease is endemic either in Hong Kong or in China as a whole."[65] The reality was that the *jiaoqi* illness had been observed and managed only by Chinese doctors in Chinese institutions up to this point. Like *kanpō* writers, Chinese doctors were seeing the reemerging *jiaoqi* endemic as a new, modern phenomenon in a changing world order. But their articulation of the "modern" character of the *jiaoqi* phenomenon was very different from that of *kanpō* writers. In the rest of this essay, I will briefly describe the explanations for the nineteenth-century *jiaoqi* epidemics in southern China that were given in Chinese medical texts, for the purpose of contrasting them with those given in the *kanpō* texts.

Jiaoqi in Nineteenth-Century Chinese Medical Texts

As already mentioned, *jiaoqi* was not a much-discussed disease in the late imperial period until the last two to three decades of the Qing dynasty. The only book worth mentioning is *Secret Jiaoqi Recipes* (*Jiaoqi mifang* 腳氣祕方), attributed to the famous Cantonese scholar-physician He Mengyao 何夢瑤 (1693–1754, *jinshi* 1730). This text was said to be in manuscript form and was not published until 1918. Unlike contemporary *kanpō* texts, this book, citing principles and recipes from medical classics on the disease, did not discuss *jiaoqi* in any contemporary social context. But similar to *kanpō* texts, and unlike most of the post-Song descriptions of *jiaoqi*, the treatise emphasized the terminal

63   Simmons 1880, 50.
64   Carpenter 2000, chap. 1; Heidhues 1992, 61–65.
65   Hunter 1905, 130.

chongxin "assault on the heart" caused by internal obstruction and did not confuse the disorder with various pains or numbness of the foot or leg. The published version of this text nonetheless contains a hint that suggests a possible epidemic situation in Guangdong in the early nineteenth century. In the postscript dated 1819, Huang Peifang 黃培芳 (early nineteenth century), another eminent Cantonese scholar, told the reader that the manuscript was given to him by monks in the White Cloud Monastery in Canton, who were famous for their expertise in treating *jiaoqi* and had successfully treated Huang himself.[66] By 1918, when the manuscript was finally printed for the first time, *jiaoqi* was clearly epidemic in Guangdong.

Three decades before the publication of He's book, the first modern Chinese medical book on *jiaoqi*, *Preliminary Words on* Jiaoqi (*Jiaoqi chuyan* 腳氣芻言), authored by a Cantonese doctor, Zeng Chaoran 曾超然, was published in 1887. The revival of Chinese medical writings on *jiaoqi* in the late Qing period seems to have happened at a particular conjuncture: rapidly growing emigration from southern China to various parts of the world, especially to Southeast Asia. Zeng observed many patients in the Tung Wah Hospital in Hong Kong, the first Chinese charitable hospital, which had been established in 1872 and where he had worked and taught since 1879. All ten medical cases of *jiaoqi* described in his book concerned young male patients, mostly intellectuals (students) or in clerical occupations in Hong Kong or overseas, with many being recent migrants from Guangdong.[67] Like *kanpō* doctors on *kakké*, Zeng perceived a leisurely lifestyle or one requiring little physical exertion to be a common feature of *jiaoqi* patients. Quoting major classical remedies, Zeng also mentioned more recent recipes using southern herbs or animals. The most revealing of all new therapeutics described in Zeng's text, however, is the Chinese version of *tenchi* 轉地 (*zhuandi*, "to change location"). Here *zhuandi* meant repatriating patients from their overseas workplace back to their native place, which was Canton for most patients in Zeng's text. Zeng claimed that most patients' conditions improved after being repatriated. Very different from the *kanpō* idea of moving the patient to dryer, high ground, the Chinese *zhuandi* therapy shows that *jiaoqi* was basically considered a migrant disease par excellence. In fact, the Tung Wah Hospital, where Zeng worked, was a key institution in the regular organization of transfers of overseas *jiaoqi* patients back to Canton. These repatriations began not later than 1903 and involved thousands of patients

---

66   He 1918, postscript, *juan* 4, 38.

67   Zeng 1887. Only one of the patients that he described was an agricultural worker.

every year being transported back to Canton from Southeast Asia, Latin America, and Hong Kong.[68]

Zeng's book could perhaps be considered part of a growing popular and local medical literature that seemed to be flourishing in China at that time: the *yanfang* 驗方 ("recipes proven by experience" tradition, as opposed to "classical" recipes, 經方) literature on diseases observed to be regional endemics in the nineteenth century, such as *jiaoqi*, plague, cholera, diphtheria, fevers, swollenness, and so on in the Guangdong region.[69] These *yanfang* and more formal medical texts on new diseases seemed to inform each other from the late nineteenth century onward, gradually forming a corpus of local medical texts that reinforced the idea that endemics could be treated more efficiently by local doctors and remedies,[70] an idea that was also promoted by *kanpō* doctors for *kakké*. Just as *kakké* was thought to be a national disease of modern Japan, *jiaoqi* in China was often described as typically "southern."[71] It is interesting to note that British doctors in Hong Kong, including Patrick Manson and James Cantlie of the tropical medicine school, were also informed by Chinese experts on such local diseases often unknown to Western doctors. They admitted that their first contact with beriberi patients was in the Alice Memorial Hospital, established in 1887 in Hong Kong as the first privately funded charitable Western hospital treating Chinese. The report on their first observations shows that they were essentially instructed by local Chinese doctors, possibly including

---

68   The Tung Wah Hospital partnered with the major charitable Chinese medical hospital in Canton, the Fangbian Hospital 方便醫院, to organize the repatriation of *jiaoqi* patients. At first, patients were transported to Canton via the West River; later in the twentieth century, they traveled on the Canton–Kowloon train. The Tung Wah Hospital, as a major charitable organization for Hong Kong and overseas Chinese since 1871, paid the Fangbian Hospital for accommodating patients repatriated by the Tung Wah. See Leung 2010.

69   Many of these popular texts were compiled and published by herbal stores in Canton, and some of these works had several editions. I have in hand an undated and anonymous text also called *Jiaoqi chuyan*, a short work that contains popular recipes. One very popular work, called *Record to Provide Relief to the Populace* (*Ji zhong lu* 濟眾錄), included short texts and recipes on plague, *jiaoqi*, cholera, fevers, and swollenness and a prayer to ask for rain. *Complete Records of the Xinggong Charitable Hall* (*Xinggong quanlu* 省躬全錄), a long manuscript on various "local" diseases published in 1914 by a Daoist charitable hall in Canton, contained pages of recipes on *jiaoqi*.

70   It is interesting to note that the recently published series of Cantonese medical texts of the late Qing and early Republican period reveal an emerging medicine with "Cantonese" characteristics. Many of the texts are on endemic diseases of the period. See Zheng 2009.

71   This point was emphasized in the reedition of Zeng's book by the Guangdong military in 1914.

Zeng, who was then employed as a doctor and teacher in the Tung Wah Hospital, on the clinical pattern, causes, and therapeutics of the disease.[72]

The revival of interest in *jiaoqi* in China was also a consequence of a growing epidemic in Shanghai, a place that Chinese doctors described as an ideal breeding ground for *jiaoqi* because of its low topography and muggy climate. Shanghai was thus similar to those insalubrious Japanese coastal cities where *kakké* was rampant. Ding Fubao 丁福保 (1874–1952), well versed in traditional medicine but also a major translator of Japanese medical texts into Chinese since 1908, published the first compilation of classical texts on *jiaoqi* with translated Japanese texts on *kakké* in 1910.[73] Translated passages revealed competing biomedical theories on beriberi: toxins in the form of mold or in fish or spoiled foods, contagion, special lifestyles of men, immobility, miasma, low standard of living, shoes that don't fit, and so on. Toxin in rice as a result of bad storage rather than something intrinsic was also mentioned as a possible cause but was not given as much weight as miasma. White rice as a cause was viewed with skepticism. Ding himself considered toxin in spoiled rice an important cause, with bad local environment (*shuitu* 水土, "water/earth") a secondary cause. He was typically eclectic in his therapeutic recommendations: observing life-nurturing principles, restraint from sexual activity, avoidance of violent exercise, attention to food, transferring the patient to higher ground, and bloodletting to release the pressure on the heart. While Ding introduced Japanese and biomedical explanations of the disease in his book, his contemporary, a much-respected traditional practitioner, Zhou Xiaonong 周小農 (1876–1942), who practiced in Shanghai until 1911, provided us with concrete medical cases of the time. These cases illustrate the rapid urbanization of Shanghai as the background of the growing epidemic, as many of his patients were immigrants to Shanghai from other parts of China. Uninformed immigrants, especially young men seeking opportunities in this big city, were described as particularly vulnerable because they were unaccustomed to the unhealthy environment and unfamiliar with the symptoms and treatment when they contracted *jiaoqi*. Like Zeng, he recommended returning to their native place as one of the most reliable treatments.[74] Modern Chinese medical writers did not seem to question the stability of the old *jiaoqi* ailment and attributed more importance to external pathogens as the key cause of the disease, as did Tang classics. However, even though they did not formulate any

---

72   Gibson 1900.

73   Ding 1910.

74   Zhou 1971, 194–202. His patients were again all male; although employed in different businesses and institutions, they obviously belonged to a middle class.

notion of the "mutability" of *jiaoqi* as did *kanpō* authors, they had little problem situating the epidemic in the modern context.

Conclusion

While both *kanpō* authors and traditional Chinese doctors of the period understood and explained *kakké* and *jiaoqi* with the same classical vocabulary, the ailment was perceived as a modern phenomenon. *Kanpō* doctors increasingly depicted *kakké* as a distinct disease of modern, urbanized, and affluent Japan. It was, above all, a "changing" disease. Chinese doctors continued to view *jiaoqi* as the disease with the same name in the medieval period and highlighted its regional nature, yet they placed it in a totally modern context of global migration: the disease was observed to affect mainly immigrants in overseas tropical regions or in major southern cities in China. Japanese and Chinese doctors elaborated on both the external and the internal causes developed by medieval and Jin and Yuan masters to explain the respective patterns of the epidemics they were observing, and they similarly concluded that the disease affected mostly young urban males of respectable social status or men with rich diets or undisciplined lifestyles. While removal of patients to high and dry ground far from city centers was a modern *kanpō* therapeutic option, Chinese doctors recommended repatriation to the patient's native place, both methods articulating clearly two different experiences and readings of the unsettling, globalizing modern world.

   Kanpō and Chinese doctors made sense of the emerging world of the nineteenth century by viewing *kakké* and *jiaoqi* as a disease category that was multicausal, as taught by the old classics, but also socially, regionally, or even ethnically bounded, which sometimes explained its changeability and how it affected mostly an up-and-coming class of respectable young men entering a competitive, alienating, and globalizing world of opportunities and risks. For a long time it was considered a disease of the privileged, not of the deprived, as implied in classical texts. Western biomedical scientists, on the other hand, observed Asian beriberi patients among laborers and coolies in plantations, prisons, asylums, camps, orphanages, and schools in the colonies. They experimented with chicken, pigeons, and other animals, which provided them with data that inspired the construction of the nutrient deficiency theory focusing on a quintessentially Asian staple food—rice—leading ultimately to the discovery and study of vitamins, *the* cutting-edge biochemical research at the turn of the twentieth century. Viewing beriberi as a new, universal, specific, and unicausal disease victimizing impoverished and ignorant Asian populations with a deficient diet consisting only of white rice was the way that nineteenth-century Western biomedical experts made sense of colonized Asia. This was completely different from *kanpō* and Chinese doctors' worldview, which was based on their everyday experience and their knowledge of classical texts, which retained their explanatory power well into the twentieth century. It is thus understandable that the theory of malnutrition caused by a diet of white rice took a long time to have any real, albeit limited impact in Asia.[75]

References

Arnold, David 1994. "The 'Discovery' of Malnutrition and Diet in Colonial India," *Indian Economic and Social History Review* 31: 1–26.

―――― 2009. "Tropical Governance: Managing Health in Monsoon Asia, 1908–1938," Asia Research Institute Working Paper no. 116, National University of Singapore, May 12.

―――― 2010. "British India and the 'Beriberi Problem,' 1798–1942," *Medical History* 54: 295–314.

The Bantam Medical Dictionary 2000. New York: Bantam Books.

Bay, Alexander 2006. "The Politics of Disease: Beriberi, Barley, and Medicine in Modern Japan (1700–1939)." Ph.D. diss., Stanford University.

Carpenter, Kenneth 2000. *Beriberi, White Rice, and Vitamin B: A Disease, a Cause, and a Cure.* Berkeley: University of California Press.

Chang, Chia-feng 2000. "Dispersing the Foetal Toxin of the Body: Conceptions of Smallpox Aetiology in Pre-modern China," in L. Conrad and D. Wujastyk, eds., *Contagion: Perspectives from Pre-modern Societies.* Aldershot, England: Ashgate, 23–38.

Ding Fubao 丁福保 1910. *Jiaoqi bing zhi yuanyin ji zhifa* 腳氣病之原因及療法 [Causes and treatment of the *jiaoqi* ailment]. Shanghai: Wenming shuju.

Gibson, R. M. 1900. "Beriberi in Hong Kong with Special Reference to the Records of the Alice Memorial and Nethersole Hospitals and with Notes on Two Years' Experience of the Disease," manuscript dated March 16, 1900.

Hanson, Marta 2011. *Speaking of Epidemics in Chinese Medicine.* London: Routledge.

He Mengyao 何夢瑤 1918. *Jiaoqi mifang* 腳氣秘方 [Secret *jiaoqi* recipes]. Guangzhou: Liangguang tushuju.

Heidhues, Mary 1992. *Bangka Tin and Mentok Pepper: Chinese Settlement on an Indonesian Island.* Singapore: Institute of Southeast Asian Studies.

Hunter, William 1905. "The Incidence of Disease in Hong Kong," *Journal of Tropical Medicine*, May 1, 130.

---

75   See Arnold 2009, 2010.

Imamura Ryō 今村亮 1861. *Kakké kōyō* 脚氣鈎要 [Essentials on *kakké*]. Edo: Keigyōkan.

——— 1878. *Kakké shinron* 脚氣新論 [New treatise on *kakké*]. Edo: Keigyōkan.

Kamminga, H., and A. Cunningham 1995. *The Science and Culture of Nutrition, 1840–1940.* Amsterdam: Rodopi.

Leung, Angela Ki Che 2010. "Understanding and Managing *Jiaoqi* in Colonial Asia, ca. 1850–1940," paper presented at the conference "The (After)Life of Traditional Knowledge," London, August 21.

Liang Qizi 梁其姿 (Leung, Angela Ki Che) 2002. "Jibing yu fangtu zhi guanxi: Yuan zhi Qing jian yijie di kanfa" 疾病與方土之關係: 元至清間醫界的法 [Disease and locality: Medical opinions between the Yuan and the Qing dynasties]. In K. Wang, ed., *Xingbie yu yiliao* 性別與醫療 [Gender and medicine], Committee of the Third International Conference on Sinology. Taibei: Academia Sinica, Institute of Modern History, 165–212.

Liao Yuqun 廖育羣 2001. "Jizai yu quanshi: Riben jiaoqi bing shi di zai jiantao" 記載與詮釋: 日本脚氣病史的再檢討 [Records and interpretations: Revisiting the history of *kakké* in Japan], *Hsin shixue* [New history] 12, 4: 121–154.

——— 2011. "Guanyu Zhongguo gudai di jiaoqi bing ji qi lishi di yanjiu" 關於中國古代的脚氣病及其歷史的研究 [The *jiaoqi* disorder in ancient China and research on its history], in F.-S. Lin, ed., *Jibing di lishi* 疾病的歷史 [The history of disease]. Taibei: Linking Publishers, 245–267.

Maruyama Genshō 丸山元璋 1811. *Kakké bensei* 脚氣辨正 [Distinguishing the correct (theories on) *kakké*]. Seikansai 靜閒齋 edition. Osaka: Torikai Ichizaemon; Kishū: Takaichi Ihē, Tanaka Heiemon.

Matsui Zaian 松井材庵 1766. *Kakké hōron* 脚氣方論 [On recipes to treat *kakké*]. Manuscript, preface by Itō Inei 伊東維寧.

Minamoto Yasunori 源養德 (1763) 1899. *Kakké ruihō* 脚氣類方 [Recipes on *kakké*]. Shanghai: Guxiangge.

Nakano Yasuaki 岡田昌春 and Asada Sōhaku 淺田惟常 (1879) 1993. *Kakké gairon* 脚氣概論 [General treatise on *kakké*], in *Huang Han yixue congzhu*, 1936. Repr., Shanghai: Zhongyi xueyuan chubanshe.

Oberlander, Christian 2005. "The Rise of Western 'Scientific Medicine' in Japan: Bacteriology and Beriberi," in Morris Low, ed., *Building a Modern Japan: Science, Technology, and Medicine in the Meiji Era and Beyond.* New York: Palgrave Macmillan, 13–36.

Okamoto Shōan 岡田昌庵 1812. *Seikei hohō kakké bunrui hen* 聖惠補方脚氣分類編 [Classified and supplemented compilation of recipes on *kakké* in the *Shenghui fang*]. Edo: Senshōbō.

Pan Guijuan 潘桂娟 and Fan Zhenglun 樊正倫 1994. *Riben Hanfang yixue* 日本漢方醫學 [*kanpō* medicine]. Beijing: Zhongguo zhongyiyao chubanshe.

Ryō Onjin 廖溫仁 1936. *Tōyō kakkebyō kenkyū* 東洋腳氣病研究 [Research on the *jiaoqi* ailment in China]. Kyoto: Kaniya shoten.

Scrinis, Gyorgy 2008. "On the Ideology of Nutritionism," *Gastronomica: The Journal of Food and Culture* 8, 1: 39–48.

Simmons, Duane 1880. "Beriberi, or the 'Kakké' of Japan," *Medical Reports, for the Half Year Ended 31st March*, nineteenth issue, China Imperial Maritime Customs, II Special Series, no. 2. Shanghai: Statistical Department of the Inspectorate General.

Smith, Hilary 2008. "Foot-qi: History of a Chinese Medical Disorder." Ph.D. diss., University of Pennsylvania.

Sun Simiao 孫思邈 (1307) 1955. *Beiji qianjin yaofang* 備急千金要方 [Essential recipes for urgent use worth a thousand gold pieces]. Beijing: Renmin weisheng chubanshe.

Tachibana Genshu 橘元周 1787. *Kakkésetsu* 腳氣說 [On *kakké*].

Taki Motokata 多紀元堅 (Tanba Genken 丹波元堅) (1853) 1983. *Zatsubyō kōyō* 雜病廣要 [Broad essentials of various diseases]. 2nd ed. Beijing: Renmin weisheng chubanshe.

Tōyama Chinkichi 遠山椿吉 1913. *Kakké yobōhō to chiryōhō* 腳氣豫防法と治療法 [Prevention and treatment of *kakké*]. Tokyo: Kōbundō.

Williams, Robert 1961. *Towards the Conquest of Beriberi.* Cambridge, MA: Harvard University Press.

Worboys, Michael 1988. "The Discovery of Colonial Malnutrition between the Wars," in David Arnold, ed., *Imperial Medicine and Indigenous Societies.* Manchester: Manchester University Press, 208–225.

Zeng Chaoran 曾超然 1887. *Jiaoqi chuyan* 腳氣芻言 [Preliminary words on *jiaoqi*]. Guangzhou: Juzhentang.

Zheng Hong 鄭洪 2009. *Lingnan yixue yu wenhua* 嶺南醫學與文化 [Medicine and culture in the Lingnan region]. Guangzhou: Guangdong keji chubanshe.

Zhou Xiaonong 周小農 1971. *Zhou Xiaonong yi'an* 周小農醫案 [Medical cases of Zhou Xiaonong]. Hong Kong: Commercial Press.

CHAPTER 9

Yang Shoujing and the Kojima Family: Collection and Publication of Medical Classics

Mayanagi Makoto, with Takashi Miura and Mathias Vigouroux

Introduction

The mid-Edo period saw the rise of the Ancient Formulas School (Kohō-ha 古方派), spearheaded by Yoshimasu Tōdō 吉益東洞 (1702–1773). This school not only reinvigorated the "Japanization" of traditional medicine but also critiqued and made corrections to Chinese medical classics on the basis of its unique interpretations. In the late Edo period, the method of Qing Evidential Studies was applied to the study of medical classics, and this led to the establishment of the School of Evidential Studies of Medicine (Kōshō igaku-ha 考證醫學派), with its center at the Edo Medical School (Edo igakukan 江戶醫學館) and many of its contributors being *bakufu* medical officials. This school began to expand its influence as a counterpart to the Ancient Formulas School.

Proponents of the School of Evidential Studies of Medicine engaged in extensive analyses of Chinese and Japanese classics and produced many works on medical texts from an empirical standpoint.[1] As the foundation for these endeavors, they edited and published many medical classics of good quality[2] and restored Chinese medical texts and pre-Tang pharmacological texts that had been lost. Many rare books and documents were collected for this purpose. Results of their analyses were the compilation of the *Iseki kō* 醫籍考 (*Investigation of Chinese Medical Books*), consisting of eighty *juan*, by Taki Mototsugu 多紀元胤 (1789–1827) in 1826 and the *Keiseki hōkoshi* 經籍訪古志 (*Bibliography of Rare Chinese Classics in Japan*), consisting of eight *juan*, by Mori Tatsuyuki 森立之 (1807–1885), Shibue Chūsai 澀江抽齋 (1805–1858),

---

1   Machi 2004; Kosoto 2004.

2   *Iryaku shō* 醫略抄, *Honzō wamyō* 本草和名 (1796); *Nan jing jizhu* 難経集注 (1804); *Shengji zonglu* 聖濟總錄 (1816); *Bencao yanyi* 本草衍義 (1823); *Hama jing* 蝦蟇經 (1823); *Qianjin yifang* 千金翼方 (1829); *Zhenben qianjinfang* 眞本千金方 (1832); *Zhujie Shanghan lun* 注解傷寒論 (1835); *Qianjin yaofang* 千金要方 (1849); *Yifang leiju* 醫方類聚 (1852–1861); *Jingui yaolue* 金匱要略 (1853); *Suwen* 素問 (1855); *Songban Shanghan lun* 宋板傷寒論 (1856); *Ishinpō* 醫心方 (1860).

and others in 1856. With these major accomplishments, the School of Evidential Studies of Medicine was at the peak of its influence on the eve of the Meiji Restoration.

Meiji Japan adopted the policy of the exclusive promotion of Western medicine. Factions in favor of traditional medicine engaged in a variety of activities to oppose this trend, but these efforts vanished completely by 1902.[3] As a result, traditional medicine in Japan lost both its foundation and its successors at this time. Works on traditional medicine, which had reached an unprecedented level of sophistication by the late Edo period, began to be circulated in antique book markets. Qing scholars and merchants who were in Japan at this time purchased some of these medical books and introduced them to China. One of them, Yang Shoujing 楊守敬 (1839–1915), who was born to a merchant family in Yidu of Hubei, pioneered this movement and bought the largest quantity of books during his stay in Japan.[4]

From his teens, Yang Shoujing aspired to reach the rank of "Presented Scholar" (*jinshi* 進士) through the imperial examination. By the age of twenty-four, he had passed the first four levels of examination (the district, prefectural, academic, and provincial examinations); however, he failed the subsequent metropolitan examination in Beijing ten years in a row. During his years in Beijing, Yang collected books in the Liulichang district of Beijing and interacted with the city's literati. Toward the end of 1879, Yang received an invitation to go to Japan from He Ruzhang 何如璋 (1838–1891), Qing China's first minister (*kōshi, gongshi* 公使) to Japan.[5] Yang arrived in Japan in 1880, after having failed the metropolitan examination one more time, and remained in Japan until 1884. During his stay there, he purchased many rare books of good quality (*zenpon, shanben* 善本).

Yang used *Keiseki hōkoshi* as a reference in searching for and collecting rare books. Mori Tatsuyuki, one of the compilers of the book, served as an intermediary for Yang.[6] Mori was a physician belonging to the School of Evidential Studies of Medicine, and he helped Yang collect many medical books. In 1884 Yang compiled and published his findings in Japan as *Guyi congshu* 古逸叢書 (*Series of Old Books Lost in China*) while still in the country. After returning to

---

3   Yakazu 1977, 1–35.

4   For full details on Yang's collection of texts, which will be analyzed in the following sections, refer to the original version of this article, Mayanagi 2008. Also see http://repository. kulib.kyoto-u.ac.jp/dspace/handle/2433/88025.

5   Wu 1974, 1–30.

6   In the introduction of Yang Shoujing's *Riben fangshu zhi*, he notes, "I ... had an association with the country's medical officer Mori Tatsuyuki and saw his work *Keiseki hōkoshi*. I eventually searched for these [books], using his work as a reference."

China, he published in 1901 a meticulous record of the books he had purchased in Japan under the title *Ribcn fangshu zhi* 日本訪書志 (*Bibliography of Old Books Obtained in Japan*). In the section titled "Yuanqi" 緣起 ("The Origin"), written in 1881, he claims that within a year of arriving in Japan, he had purchased over 30,000 *juan* and that many of these were old texts formerly owned by physicians.[7] He also writes that he obtained the majority of medical books from members of the Kojima family—namely, Naokata 尚質, Naomasa 尚眞, and Shōkei 尚絅. There are no documents that corroborate the exact number of books Yang purchased in Japan or the background of how he obtained them. It is possible to gain insight, however, by turning our attention to the Kojima family, who have not received much academic attention thus far.

Moreover, in the past, scholars have done much to analyze the relationship between Yang and Mori. However, not enough attention has been given to Yang's publication of medical texts and his motives in doing so. The goal of this essay is to shed light upon these hitherto-neglected points. By doing so, we can learn how the knowledge of collation and revision from *bakumatsu* Japan was transmitted to China and how it impacted scholarship and publishing in the late Qing period.

The Kojima Family's Scholarship and Collection

Scholarship

The progenitor of the Kojima family was named Ensai 圓齋 (?–1657). He was appointed in 1648 to the position of *oku ishi* 奧醫師 (in-house medical officer for the Tokugawa shogun and his family). His descendants inherited the position as *bakufu* medical officials until the end of the Tokugawa regime during the time of the tenth-generation head of the household, Shōkei.

The eighth-generation head of the household, Naokata (1797–1848), had the Chinese-style name (*azana* 字) of Gakko 學古 and the pen name (*gō* 號) of Hōso 寶素. He began his study at the Edo Medical School at an early age, became *ban'i* 番醫 (the highest-ranking medical officer attending to *bakufu* bureaucrats) at the age of twenty-five, obtained the ranks of *hōgen* 法眼 (the second-highest rank bestowed upon a medical officer) and *oku ishi* at forty-five, and was appointed *igakukan sewayaku* 醫學館世話役 (supervisor) at fifty. He died at the age of fifty-two. Naokata excelled in the collation of medical books, and his work was continued by his sons Naomasa and Shōkei. The work of text collation involves searching for identical or similar contents in old

---

7   Yang (1901) 1967.

texts and analyzing the reasons for similarities and differences. Text collation is useful for understanding the lineage of a particular text as well as the relationship between the original and its copies.

The ninth-generation head of the household, the third son of Naokata, was Naomasa (1829–1857), with the Chinese name of Hōchū 抱沖, the common name of Shunki 春沂, and the pen name of Shōin 椶蔭. At the age of eleven, he became a disciple of Taki Motokata 多紀元堅 (1795–1857) and, from then on, participated in a study group hosted by Naokata on *Qianjin yifang* 千金翼方 (*Recipes Worth a Thousand Gold Pieces*). At the age of seventeen, he was appointed *sodoku yaku* 素讀役 (reader) at the Edo Medical School, and at twenty-one, he became the head of the Kojima family and was also appointed *ban'i*. At the age of twenty-five, he was appointed *igakukan sewayaku*, and at twenty-six, *yoriai ishi* 寄合醫師 (the second-highest medical officer for bureaucrats). He died at the age of twenty-nine. The collation work of Naokata and Naomasa resulted in Naomasa's *Iseki choroku* 醫籍著錄 (*Catalog of Chinese Medical Books*; now in the collection of the National Palace Museum 故宮博物院 in Taibei) and is also reflected in various sections of *Keiseki hōkoshi*.

The tenth-generation head of the household, the fourth son of Naokata, was Shōkei (1839–1880), with the Chinese name of Tanki 瞻淇 and the pen name of Shikin 子錦. He inherited the household by being adopted by his childless older brother Naomasa. At the age of eighteen, he began to live in the dormitory of the Edo Medical School (*igakukan kishukuryō* 醫學館寄宿寮). He became head of the household when he was twenty and was appointed *kishukuryō tōdori yaku* 寄宿寮頭取役 (director of the dormitory) at the age of twenty-four and *sewayaku* of the dormitory at the age of twenty-nine. He lost his official post after the Meiji Restoration and died when he was forty-two. The room in which the Kojima family's texts were kept during these three generations was called Hōso-dō 寶素堂 (the Hall of Hōso).

Collection

We can get a glimpse of the Kojima family's collection by looking at *Hōso-dō zōsho mokuroku* 寶素堂藏書目錄 (*Catalog of the Book Collection in the Hall of Hōso*), edited by Naomasa. The catalog offers information exclusively on Chinese medical texts, including their titles, the number of *juan*, and their bibliographic records—522 titles in total. Of the texts cataloged, the number of medical texts from the Song period is the highest by far. The majority of the texts in the catalog are of good quality. It is highly unlikely, however, that the Kojima family's collection consisted exclusively of quality texts. It is safe to say that more than half of the family's collection, including those texts not included in the catalog, consisted of old texts of average quality. If we accept this estimation, then it follows that the Kojima family's entire collection contained more than 1,000 titles, counting just Chinese texts.

Furthermore, in *Kōkoku iseki mokuroku* 皇國醫籍目錄 (*Catalog of Japanese Medical Books*), Naomasa records 78 rare medical texts of good quality from or predating the Keichō period (1596–1614). Approximately half of the Kojima family's collection is now stored in the National Palace Museum in Taibei, for reasons that will be explained below. In the National Palace Museum, 35 Japanese titles on medicine are identified as originally belonging to the Kojima family, including 5 written by members of the family. Those not written by members of the Kojima family mostly match the records found in *Kōkoku iseki mokuroku*. The museum also has 147 Chinese titles formerly belonging to the Kojima family, including 14 titles on medicine. If one were to do a simple calculation based on the ratio between the numbers of Japanese and Chinese titles in the museum and the number of texts in the Chinese collection as recorded in *Hōso-dō zōsho mokuroku* ($147/35 = 522/x$), then the number of Japanese titles on medicine that the Kojima family owned can be estimated at 124. However, just as with the collection of Chinese texts, the Kojima family most likely did not exclusively collect quality texts related to medicine. If we take this into consideration, the number of Japanese texts held by the Kojima family, including those on medicine, can be estimated roughly at around 300 titles at the very least.

Given these estimates, the Kojima family probably held at least 646 rare medical texts of quality from China and Japan. If one were to include average-quality texts into the count, the Kojima family's collection would exceed 1,000 Chinese titles and would include at least 300 Japanese titles. Since the Taki family's *Seijukan iseki bikō* 躋壽館醫籍備考 (*Remarks on Medical Books at Seijukan*, 1877) records 1,390 titles on medicine,[8] it is not farfetched to estimate that the Kojima family's collection, including texts not related to medicine, was around 1,300 titles. I use "title" to mean one complete piece of work, which can consist of multiple *juan*. A title may consist of one *juan* or maybe even forty *juan*. If one were to convert 1,300 titles into the number of *juan*, the number would definitely be in the several thousands, perhaps as high as 5,000. In Japan's Cabinet Library 內閣文庫, one of the best archives in the world of rare Chinese medical texts of good quality, there are 1,632 pre-Qing Chinese medical titles.[9] From this number alone, one can appreciate the scale of the Kojima family's collection.

---

8   Mori Junzaburō 1985, 276.
9   Mayanagi and Wang 1998.

Old Medical Books Obtained by Yang Shoujing in Japan

Obtaining Books from the Kojima Family

Yang arrived in Japan in April 1880 at the age of forty-two and returned home in May 1884.[10] As already mentioned, he claims to have collected over 30,000 *juan* in less than a year and that many of the rare medical texts he obtained came from the Kojima family's collection. Why was he able to obtain so many books from the Kojima family? The last of the three generations of the Kojima family discussed above, Shōkei, lost his official position after the Meiji Restoration and died on December 5, 1880.[11] Yang had arrived in Japan in April of the same year. Under the entry on *Waitai miyao fang* 外臺祕要方 (*Medical Secrets from the Royal Library*) in *Riben fangshu zhi*, Yang writes, "Following the advice of Mori Tatsuyuki, I first purchased this book on which Kojima Gakko [i.e., Naokata] had written notes concerning variations between texts."[12] It is not clear, however, exactly when Mori recommended that Yang purchase Naokata's *Waitai*. This information is also not available for *Shinkyaku hitsuwa* 清客筆話 (*Conversations through Writing with a Guest from the Qing*), a record of written communications between Mori and Yang. *Shinkyaku hitsuwa* begins with an entry on January 21, 1881, and Yang's business card is pasted into the text at this entry.[13] Yang and Mori probably met for the first time on this day, and Mori most likely introduced Yang to the Kojima family's collection sometime after this. Yang thus became aware of the Kojima family's large collection of quality books and eventually purchased many of them.

Obtaining Books from Sources Other Than the Kojima Family

The medical texts that Yang purchased in Japan were not limited to those of the Kojima family. As evident in *Riben fangshu zhi*, Yang purchased books from a number of families. After Yang's death, the majority of his collection was purchased by the government of the Republic of China. Today, these books can be found at the National Palace Museum in Taibei and the National Library of China 中國國家圖書館 in Beijing.

I have examined the entirety of Yang's collection that can be found in the National Palace Museum. Based on the ownership stamps and handwritten notes left in the books, I was able to figure out where these books had come from. In order of quantity, books in Yang's collection had come from (1) the

---

10   Wu 1974, 30.
11   Mori Rintarō 1979, 360.
12   Yang (1901) 1967, 654.
13   Ishida 1990.

Kojima family, (2) the Edo Medical School and the Taki family, (3) individuals affiliated with the Edo Medical School, and (4) others. As already mentioned, the Kojima family probably held at least 646 rare medical books from China and Japan. Yang most likely purchased the majority of them. At the National Palace Museum, 169 medical books can be identified as having originally come from the Kojima family. These books constitute roughly 37 percent of the collection of old medical books formerly belonging to Yang (451 titles). Based on a simple calculation (169/451 = 646/x), it can be estimated that Yang purchased 1,724 old medical books in Japan. Thus, a very large quantity of old medical books, possibly comparable to the holdings of the Cabinet Library, moved from Japan to China with Yang.

Yang Shoujing's Publication of Medical Books

Yang edited and published many books, including *Guyi congshu*, *Riben fangshu zhi*, *Liuzhen pu* 留眞譜 (*Facsimile of Rare Books*), and *Shui jing zhu* 水經注 (*Commentary on the Waterways Classic*). Wu Tianren and Zhao Feipeng compiled catalogs of Yang's publications, but the only medical title covered in the catalogs is *Daguan bencao* 大觀本草 (*Materia Medica of the Daguan Period*).[14] Chen Jie mentioned Yang's involvement in the publication of *Bencao yanyi* 本草衍義 (*Augmented Materia Medica*), *Shanghan lun* 傷寒論 (*Treatise on Cold Damage Disorders*), and *Maijing* 脈經 (*Classic of Pulse Diagnosis*).[15] Yang was involved in the publication of other medical books as well; however, the background of these publication activities and Yang's motives in carrying them out have not been discussed extensively. What follows is an examination of Yang's contributions to the publication of individual medical books.

Reprinting of Books Related to the Taki Family

After returning to China, Yang headed to Huanggang to work as a teacher in June 1884 and most likely began teaching in July. In August, using woodblocks purchased in Japan, he reprinted some works of the Taki family—thirteen titles, consisting of seventy *juan*—as *Yuxiu Tang yixue congshu* 聿修堂醫學叢書 (*Medical Series of Yuxiu Tang*). The introduction to this series notes, "Taki Motoyasu 多紀元簡 and his sons are authorities of Japanese medicine. The documents in this series demonstrate their erudition. Even in China, there

---

14   Wu 1974, 1–12; Zhao 1991, 45–63.

15   Chen 2003, 532–536.

have not been many physicians who can match them since the time of the Yuan dynasty."

There is an entry for December 19, 1882, in *Shinkyaku hitsuwa* concerning Yang's purchase of the woodblocks.[16] The Taki family, who for generations had presided over the Edo Medical School as *bakufu* medical officials, lost all their official positions due to the Meiji Restoration and even had to let go of their woodblocks for book production, the very embodiment of generations of family scholarship. Thanks to Yang's reprinting in China as *Yuxiu Tang yixue congshu*, however, the Taki family's scholarship was transmitted to later generations. The publication of this series was the beginning of a systematic introduction of Japanese scholarship on traditional medicine to China. After this, many scholarly works on traditional medicine from Japan, including works not belonging to the Evidential Studies tradition, were published in China. Furthermore, with the publication of *Keiseki hōkoshi* in 1885 and *Riben fangshu zhi* in 1901, Chinese intellectuals became increasingly aware of the existence of numerous rare books of good quality in Japan, later resulting in many Chinese visitors to Japan looking for and purchasing these rare texts.

Collation and Publication of Maijing 脈經

In 1893, Yang published *Maijing*, comprising ten *juan*. In the introduction, Yang lists various editions of *Maijing* since the Song period and stresses the rarity of quality editions. He furthermore explains that he purchased in Japan a Southern Song He Daren 何大任 edition from 1217 as well as editions from the Yuan and Ming periods and that he collated them and published the result as his *Maijing*. However, according to *Keiseki hōkoshi* and *Iseki choroku*, He Daren's Song edition did not exist in Japan, and the only edition available in Japan was a facsimile of a He Daren edition from the Ming period, kept at Kaisen kaku 懷仙閣 (formerly called Yō'an in 養安院) and several other places (fig. 1). In addition, at the end of *juan* 6 of Yang's *Maijing*, it says, in accordance with the original, "kept at Yō'an in" (*Yō'an in zōsho* 養安院藏書). Therefore, the Song period He Daren edition Yang claimed to have obtained was actually the Ming facsimile from Kaisen kaku. Since Yang held both *Keiseki hōkoshi* and *Iseki choroku* in his possession, he was undoubtedly aware of the two documents' assessment of the Kaisen kaku edition as a Ming replication. Nonetheless, Yang still claimed that he used a He Daren edition from the Song period as the source text for his publication. In the title and introduction, he presents his work as a facsimile of the Song edition (*ying Song* 景 (影) 宋).

---

16   Chen 1997, 538.

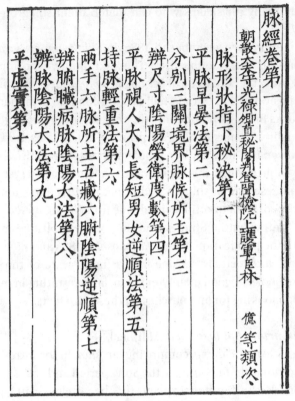

FIGURE 1   *The Ming facsimile of the He Daren edition of*
Maijing. *Neither character count nor worker's*
name is given at the center of the woodblock.
(*Book number 10-63, Seikadō Bunko, Tokyo*)

There are other questionable points concerning Yang's *Maijing*. On many
pages in Yang's edition, one can find a character count at the top of the center
of the woodblock and the woodcut worker's name at the bottom (fig. 2). But in
the Ming facsimile, there are no such indications. Does this mean that Yang did
after all use the genuine Song He Daren edition and faithfully recorded the information found in it? Workers' names recorded in Yang's edition are mostly
one-character names. Of these, only Wen 文, Lin 林, and Lü 呂 are listed in
Kegong renmin suoyin 刻工人名索引 (*Index of Woodcut Workers' Names*) by
Wang Zhongmin 王重民.[17] Many workers' names from the Song consist of two
to three characters, including surnames. Therefore, if Yang had used the Song
edition, it is unlikely that his edition would contain mostly one-character
names. At the end of the Yang edition, it is recorded, "Worked on by Tao Zilin

---

17   Wang 1983, Supplement, 100–104.

of Sanfoge, E Province" (*E sheng* [Wuhan] *Sanfoge / Tao Zilin chengke* 鄂省 [武漢] 三佛閣／陶子麟承刻). It is likely that the names Lin 林 and Lin 麟 refer to Tao Zilin 陶子麟 (林) and that other names found in the edition refer to workers at his shop. No index of woodcut workers was available when Yang's *Maijing* was published as a facsimile of the Song edition. Given this, it is reasonable to presume that Yang purposely added the workers' names and character counts, which are not recorded in the Ming facsimile of the He Daren edition, knowing full well that such manipulations would mislead people into thinking that he had used the Song He Daren edition as the source text.

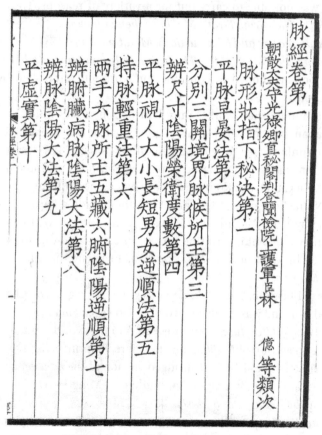

FIGURE 2   *The Yang edition of* Maijing. *The character count and the worker's name are recorded at the top and bottom of the center of the woodblock. (Book number 21513, National Library of China, Beijing)*

Why did Yang publish *Maijing* with such manipulations? Here it should be recalled that Yang interacted frequently with Mori and obtained books formerly belonging to the Taki and Kojima families. It is possible that, after purchasing so many of the two families' books, Yang had come to identify himself as an inheritor of their tradition of scholarship. In his *Riben fangshu zhi*, Yang offers many words of praise for the Taki and Kojima families. Through his writing, Yang also engages actively with bygone scholars of the two families, at times seeming to want to emulate them and at other times to refute them. Members of the Taki and Kojima families once worked at the Edo Medical School and carried out numerous projects, including collation and publication of reliable medical books (such as those mentioned in note 2). However, there were projects on quality pre-Tang and Tang medical books that the Edo Medical School was not able to carry out for a variety of reasons. These included *Lingshu* 靈樞 (*The Divine Pivot*), *Maijing*, *Zhenjiu jiayi jing* 鍼灸甲乙經 (*The Classic of Acupuncture and Moxibustion*), *Mingtang jing* 明堂經 (*The Classic of the Luminous Hall*), *Taisu* 太素 (*The Ultimate Foundation*), and *Waitai miyao fang*. Yang perhaps hoped to continue the work left unfinished by the Edo Medical School.

Of these unpublished works, Yang had obtained facsimiles of *Taisu* and *Waitai* in Japan, both of which were of good quality. However, these two titles were too voluminous for Yang to publish all by himself. Two less-voluminous books that Yang had also purchased were *Mingtang jing* and *Maijing*. *Mingtang jing* was lost in China, but Kojima Naokata had copied it from a facsimile preserved at Ninna Temple 仁和寺, and Yang then made a copy of this Kojima edition held by Mori. According to Chen, Yang had prepared *Mingtang jing* for publication by 1891, but its printing was never completed due to the 1911 revolution.[18] After his work on *Mingtang jing*, Yang turned to the collation and publication of *Maijing*.

After its publication, Yang's *Maijing* was generally regarded as a facsimile of the Song edition and was received favorably. However, *Sibu congkan* 四部叢刊 (*Four Branches of Literature*) soon presented to the world a photographic reprint of a Yuan edition of *Maijing*. Furthermore, Renmin weisheng chubanshe 人民衛生出版社 published an abridged version of the *Sibu congkan* edition, and in Japan also, a photographic facsimile of a Ming He Daren edition was produced in *Tōyō igaku zenpon sōsho* 東洋醫學善本叢書 (*Series of Rare Eastern Medicine Books*), published in 1981. Because of these developments, Yang's *Maijing* was reduced to obscurity, and its publication process has been left unanalyzed.

---

18   Chen 2001.

Yang's Contribution to the Publication of Wuchang yiguan congshu 武昌醫館叢書

Besides publishing books on his own, Yang was also involved in the publication of eight titles in *Wuchang yiguan congshu* (*Series of the Wuchang Medical School*), edited by Ke Fengshi 柯逢時 (1845–1912). Ke was a collector of books and had an association with Yang, who had moved to Wuchang in 1899. Given Yang's knowledge of the Edo Medical School's scholarship and publication of rare books, he must have offered helpful advice to Ke concerning the curriculum at Wuchang Medical School and its publication of medical books. There were many medical books of quality and rarity other than *Mingtang jing* and *Maijing* in Yang's possession that were worthy of publication and recognition in China. Ke was an individual with much political and financial power, and Yang assisted his publication activities perhaps with the hope that one day Ke would help him publish his own books. The following eight titles were published one after another by Wuchang Medical School under Ke's leadership and with his financial support:

1904 1. *Daguan bencao* 大觀本草 (*Materia Medica of the Daguan Period*)
1910 2. *Daguan bencao zhaji* 大觀本草札記 (*Record of the Collation of Daguan bencao*)
      3. *Bencao yanyi* 本草衍義 (*Augmented Materia Medica*)
1911 4. *Shanghan buwang lun* 傷寒補亡論 (*Treatise on Replenishment and Depletion in Cold Damage Disorders*)
      5. *Huoyou xinshu* 活幼心書 (*A Book for the Vitality of the Young*)
1912 6. *Shanghan zongbing lun* 傷寒總病論 (*Comprehensive Treatise on Cold Damage Disorders*)
      7. *Shanghan lun* 傷寒論 (*Treatise on Cold Damage Disorders*)
      8. *Shanghan baiwen ge* 傷寒百問歌 (*Poetry of a Hundred Inquiries on Cold Damage Disorders*)

Numbers 1, 3, 6, and 7 were printed imitating the character style of the Song and Yuan periods. At the end of *juan* 19 of number 3, "worked on by Tao Zilin" (*Tao Zilin qinkan* 陶子麟鋟刊) is recorded; it is likely that the group of workers led by Tao Zilin in Wuhan worked on many of these texts, as they did on Yang's *Mingtang jing* and *Maijing*. What follows is an analysis of the publication of numbers 1, 2, 3, and 7, to which Yang contributed in various ways.

Jingshi zhenglei daguan bencao 經史證類大觀本草 and *Daguan bencao zhaji* 大觀本草札記

In this edition of *Daguan bencao*, consisting of thirty-one *juan*, there is an introduction written by Ke Fengshi, but no information is given here as to the dating of the source text. On the other hand, in *Daguan bencao zhaji*, in two *juan*, there is an introduction by Ke dated June 1910, and from this, the following points can be extracted. Yang provided Ke with a facsimile of *Daguan bencao* sometime around 1901. Ke published it preliminarily in 1904 and added an introduction to it. However, there were problematic characters and phrases in this first edition. These errors were corrected, and the second edition was published in 1910 along with *Zhaji*, which explains why and how the corrections were made (fig. 3). *Zhaji* not only points out the differences in characters and phrases between the two editions but also explains that some revisions were made to the original after the differences were evaluated. Many of the revisions are based on *Zhenghe bencao* 政和本草 (*Revised Materia Medica of the Zhenghe Period*), but some are also based on the Chosŏn edition of *Daguan* and *Xinxiu bencao* 新修本草 (*Revised Materia Medica of the Tang Dynasty*) in Japan.

Ke's *Daguan bencao*, with an official seal in red ink, can be found today in the National Palace Museum in Taibei. This document is filled with Yang's detailed revisions and corrections written with a brush. As the basis for his revisions, Yang cites various medical classics and also some collated works by Japanese writers. One work Yang relies on heavily is a Wanli edition of *Zhenglei bencao* 證類本草 (*Revised Materia Medica of the Ming Dynasty*), which can also be found in the National Palace Museum. In this book, there are handwritten notes by Kojima Naokata and others from 1814 based on collation works with a Yuan edition of *Daguan bencao*. Ke notes that he borrowed facsimiles of several texts from Yang, and from this, it can also be surmised that Ke borrowed from Yang the Chosŏn edition of *Daguan* and *Xinxiu* that he used for *Zhaji*. As is clear from the above, however, Yang did much more than just lend texts; he actively contributed to Ke's publishing endeavors in various capacities, including collation.

In *Zhaji*'s "explanatory notes" (*hanrei* 凡例), Ke comments on the source text of a facsimile provided by Yang: "In the beginning section of the Zongwen shuyuan 宗文書院刊 edition from Yuan, Dade 6 (大德 6 年, 1302), there is a colophon frame (*muji* 木記).... This book [borrowed from Yang] has the same typeface and format as the Dade edition but does not have Zongwen shuyuan's colophon frame following the introduction. Its imprint is especially beautiful. I use this as the source text." This facsimile can be found today in the National Library in Taibei (fig. 4). It contains an introductory remark by Yang dated 1913, which goes as follows: "This edition, which lacks the colophon frame as seen in

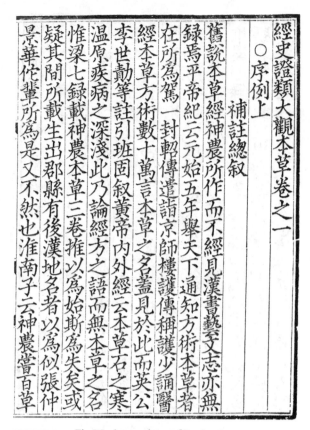

FIGURE 3   *The Wuchang edition of* Daguan bencao,
Wuchang yiguan congshu (*Beijing: Zhongguo
shudian, 1980*). (*Owned by Mayanagi*)

the Zongwen shuyuan edition, is from the Southern Song period. Zongwen shuyuan made a facsimile of this Southern Song edition during the Yuan period, and at that time, Zongwen shuyuan's colophon frame was added in the back of the margin of the introduction." I have analyzed this document firsthand to assess Yang's claim and found that it is not the case that there is no colophon frame in the back of the margin of the introduction in Yang's edition; rather, the entire backside has been ripped off. On the basis of its format and typeface, there is no doubt that this document is actually a Zongwen shuyan edition from the Yuan.

Judging from his comment above on how beautiful its imprint is, we can assume that Ke had looked at this document firsthand. It can also be inferred, from an account recorded in *Shizai Tang zayi* 世載堂雜憶 (Memories of *Shizai*

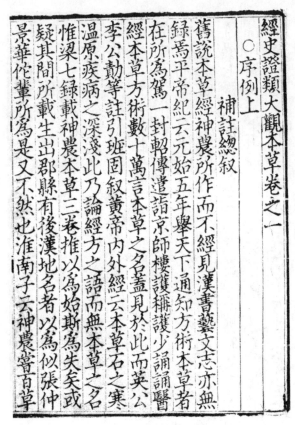

FIGURE 4   *The Yuan Dade edition of* Daguan bencao. (*Book
                 number 06212, National Central Library, Taibei*)

Tang), that Ke knew that Yang presented the document as a Song edition.[19] In
his explanatory notes, however, Ke does not admit that the text is from the
Song but says only that "I use this as the source text." This is most likely because
he did not believe Yang's claim that the document was from the Song period.
The Ke edition of *Daguan* was published as a collated facsimile of the Yuan
edition, along with detailed commentaries in *Zhaji*. The accuracy of the Ke edition becomes evident when compared with the edition available in the National Library. Ke's *Daguan, Zhaji,* and *Bencao yanyi* (as will be discussed
below) were reproduced in photographs and published together in Japan.[20] An
impetus behind this was that many regarded Ke's publications as complement-
ing the Mongolian edition of *Zhenghe bencao* (held at the National Library of

19   Liu 1960, 84–85.
20   Kimura and Yoshizaki 1970.

China, printed by Renmin Weisheng chubanshe) and hoped to read them together side by side.

Bencao yanyi 本草衍義

This work, consisting of twenty *juan*, was published in 1910 (fig. 5). In its afterword, Ke mentions two documents he received from Yang. The first document contained Yang's handwritten notes discussing similarities and differences between the Qingyuan 1 (1195) edition of *Yanyi* from the Southern Song and *Tuzhu bencao* 圖注本草 (*Materia Medica with Illustrations and Annotations*). The Qingyuan edition of *Yanyi* is mentioned in *Hōkoshi*. Yang had borrowed this document while in Japan and had compared it with *Tuzhu bencao* (the Qingyuan edition is now held by the Imperial Household Agency). The second document is a Yuan edition of *Yanyi*. Ke writes that this Yuan edition is similar in style and format to the already-published *Daguan*. He also writes that in carrying out the collation work for this document, he compared characters and phrases from different editions and also referred to Yang's handwritten notes mentioned above. In "records of collation" (*jiaoji* 校記), Ke lists key characters and phrases from different editions for each *juan* and the table of contents. From the afterword and "records of collation," it is evident that Ke relied heavily on Yang's advice and materials provided by him.

Yang's Yuan edition of *Yanyi* that matches the Wuchang edition can be found in the National Library in Taibei (fig. 6). The library catalog describes the document as "a Yuan facsimile based on the Xuanhe 1 宣和元年 (1119) edition from the Song." Characteristics of this Yuan edition are well reflected in the Wuchang edition. This Yuan edition contains an introductory remark by Yang dated 1887. However, in Yang's *Riben fangshu zhi*, there is only one entry on *Yanyi*, and it is recorded as "a Song edition." This entry on *Yanyi* in *Fangshu zhi* is identical with Yang's introductory remark in the Yuan edition, save for a few phrases. In other words, Yang wrote the introductory remark in 1887 and copied it for *Fangshu zhi*, which was published in 1901, describing his *Yanyi* as a Song edition. Since Ke published a facsimile of the Yuan edition in 1910, it is likely that Ke had obtained the document from Yang several years earlier. It goes without saying that Ke had also read *Fangshu zhi*. What this means is that in presenting his *Yanyi* to Ke, Yang withdrew his claim that it was a Song edition—as had been argued in his own work—and admitted that it was a less-prestigious Yuan edition. This was a rather self-demeaning gesture on the part of Yang. Yang and Ke were both renowned text collectors in Wuchang, but there was a significant difference between them in their social status and financial power. Forgoing his ego, Yang relied on Ke's high social standing in order to achieve his objective of publishing the books he had collected.

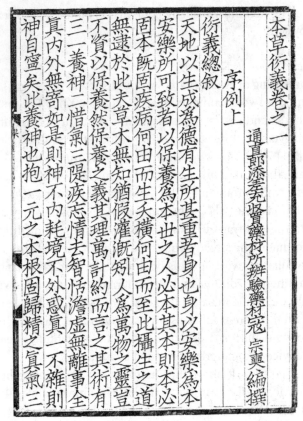

FIGURE 5   *The Wuchang edition of* Bencao yanyi, Wuchang
yiguan congshu (*Beijing: Zhongguo shudian,*
1980). (*Owned by Mayanagi*)

In the National Palace Museum in Taibei, there is a *Daguan* that formerly belonged to Yang (Case Number 64). It is cataloged as "Published by Zongwen shuyuan in Yuan, Dade 6." In reality, however, this document is an early Ming facsimile of the Zongwen shuyuan edition. In this document, one can find Kojima Naomasa's ownership stamp and Yang's handwritten introductory remark from 1885. Save for the last forty-seven characters, this introductory remark is almost identical with the one found in *Riben fangshu zhi*, which introduces the text as a Yuan document. The forty-seven characters, deleted in *Fangshu zhi*, say, "When reproducing the Northern Song *Daguan* based on this Yuan edition [in reality, a Ming facsimile], it would be ideal to also publish together with it my Song edition *Yanyi* [in reality, a Yuan edition]." Two years after this, at the end of the introductory remark to what he calls the "Song-edition" *Yanyi* (in the

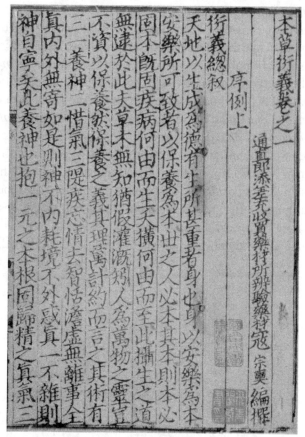

FIGURE 6   *The Yuan edition of* Bencao yanyi. *(Book number*
o62n, National Central Library, Taibei)

National Library in Taibei, the abovementioned Yuan edition), he wrote, "Because *Yanyi* was never published during the Ming dynasty, it does not appear in *Siku tiyao* 四庫提要 [*Annotated Catalog of the Imperial Library*]. Therefore, this work must be made known quickly."

As mentioned above, Ke made corrections to the first *Daguan* he published and also compiled detailed commentaries on these corrections as *Zhaji*. This can be understood as an attempt to reproduce the Northern Song *Daguan*, as described by Yang. *Yanyi* was published in 1910, the same year that Ke's second version of *Daguan* was published along with *Zhaji*. Yang's goal of collating and publishing the rare books of good quality he had obtained in Japan and of introducing them to China was thus accomplished.

Shanghan lun 傷寒論

This *Shanghan lun*, consisting of ten *juan*, was published in 1912 by Wuchang Yiguan (fig. 7). In it, one finds no commentary by Cheng Wuji 成無己 or others but finds the order of publication for a large-letter edition of *Shanghan lun* in Zhipin 2 of the Northern Song (1065) and one for a small-letter edition in Yuan-you 3 (1088). Orders of publication identical with the above two can also be found in *Songban Shanghan lun* 宋板傷寒論 (*Song Edition Treatise on Cold Damage Disorders*) in *Zhongjing quanshu* 仲景全書 (*Zhongjing's Complete Works*), which was published in 1599 during the Ming period with a foreword by Zhao Kaimei 趙開美. However, the Zhao Kaimei edition and the Wuchang edition are significantly different in format and typeface. The typeface of the Wuchang edition is in the style of the Song period and closely resembles the typeface of Yang's *Maijing*. The only existing edition of *Shanghan lun* with these particular characteristics is the Wuchang edition. On the other hand, in

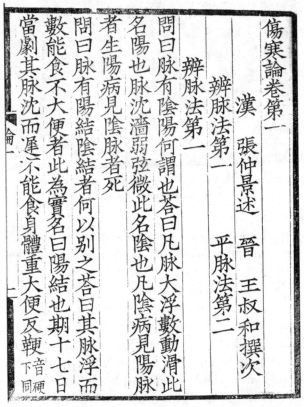

FIGURE 7   *The Wuchang edition of* Shanghan lun, Wuchang
yiguan congshu (*Beijing: Zhongguo shudian, 1980*).
(*Owned by Mayanagi*)

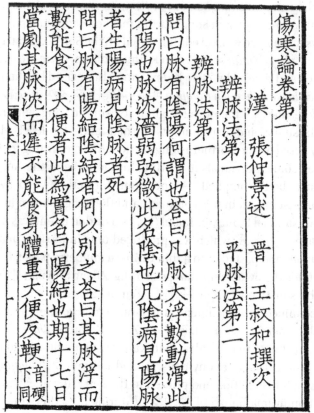

FIGURE 8　*A document that Yang claimed to be a facsimile of the*
Northern Song edition of Shanghan lun (*printed in*
Liuzhen pu chubian [*Taibei: Guangwen shuju,* 1972])

Yang's *Liuzhen pu*, published in 1901, one finds a photograph of *Shanghan lun*
(fig. 8) that closely resembles the Wuchang edition.[21] The only difference is
that in the Wuchang edition, the center of the woodcut is black, while in *Liu-*
zhen pu, it is white. Furthermore, Yang's *Fangshu zhi*, published in the same
year, refers to a document presented as "*Shanghan lun*, ten *juan*, a facsimile of
the Northern Song edition." The two orders of publication mentioned above
are also inserted in the second half of the bibliographic remark on this work.[22]

The format Yang describes in his bibliographic remark on what he calls "a
facsimile of the Northern Song edition" matches the format of the Wuchang
edition and the edition shown in the abovementioned photograph in *Liuzhen*

21　Yang (1901) 1972, 643.

22　Yang (1901) 1967, 603–615.

pu. Under the entry on *Shanghan lun* in *Fangshu zhi*, Yang claims, "I obtained this facsimile of the Northern Song edition in a bookstore in Japan. According to my analysis, the Zhao Kaimei edition relied on the Song edition. However, at the beginning of each *juan* of the Zhao Kaimei edition, there are two lines that say, 'engraved and revised by Zhao Kaimei and also revised by Shen Lin' (*Ming Zhao Kaimei jiaoke / Shen Lin tongjiao* 明趙開美校刻／沈琳全校). This edition, therefore, does not follow the original style of the Song edition. Nonetheless, this facsimile, judging from its format and the level of detail, is doubtlessly based on the Northern Song edition. After returning to the country, I encouraged some individuals to reprint this facsimile of the Northern Song edition, but nobody complied." A document formerly owned by Yang that matches the description in this comment and the image shown in *Liuzhen pu* is now in the National Library in Taibei (fig. 9). The document was handwritten on *gampi* paper 雁皮紙, which was produced only in Japan. Then the entire text was cut out and pasted onto a thin Chinese mulberry paper. On the document, one finds the ownership stamps of Yang, Zhang Shiyuan 張適園 (1872–1927), and his son Zhang Qinpu 張菦圃 (1891–1942).

I have examined this document in person, and according to my investigation, the document is clearly based on Zhao Kaimei's *Zhongjing quanshu*. However, I must note that besides Zhao Kaimei's first edition and revised edition, there also exists an anonymous pirated edition of *Zhongjing quanshu*, based on Zhao's first edition and printed in the late Ming or early Qing period (held by Momijiyama bunko 紅葉山文庫 during the Edo period and by the Cabinet Library today; fig. 10).[23] Furthermore, there is also *Sōbon shōkan ron* 宋本傷寒論 (*Song Edition Treatise on Cold Damage Disorders*), an 1856 facsimile published by Horikawa Imanari 堀川未濟—a student of Taki Motokata's—based on Momijiyama bunko's pirated *Songban Shanghan lun*. This Horikawa edition corrects errors in the pirated edition. Comparing Yang's cut-and-paste book with the editions above, the only edition that completely matches the cut-and-paste book is the pirated edition. Judging from its paper quality and scripts, the cut-and-paste edition was most likely copied by a calligrapher toward the end of the Tokugawa period. Because it was copied not from the published Horikawa edition but from the *bakufu*'s Momijiyama bunko edition, which was not available to the general public, the copy must have belonged to an individual who had influence within the Edo Medical School circle. Relating to this, in the National Palace Museum in Taibei, there is a document that is most likely a Japanese copy of *Jingui yaolue* (*Synopsis of Golden Chamber*) based on the pirated *Zhongjing quanshu* (Case Number 503). This copy was

---

23   Mayanagi 2006.

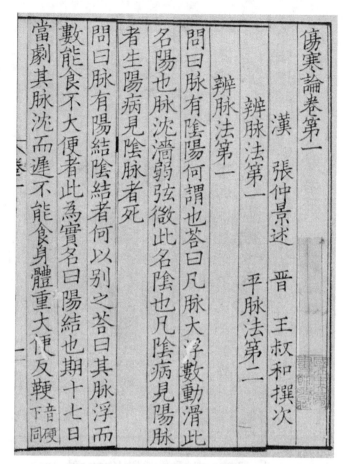

FIGURE 9   *The cut-and-paste edition of* Shanghan lun *(Book number 05895, National Central Library, Taibei)*

also made by a calligrapher on *gampi* paper. This *Jingui* contains a remark by Kojima Naomasa from 1855 and his commentaries pointing out the calligrapher's miscopies. Given this, it is not much of a stretch to imagine that Naomasa also had *Songban Shanghan lun* in the pirated *Zhongjing quanshu* copied. If we hypothesize further that the corrections of miscopies in the margins of Yang's cut-and-paste edition were also left by Naomasa, then we can conclude that Yang's cut-and-paste edition was based on the *Songban Shanghan lun* that Naomasa had copied and stored.

As mentioned above, Yang once wrote that the two lines "engraved and revised by Zhao Kaimei" and "also revised by Shen Lin" found in the Zhao Kaimei edition were evidence that this edition was not made in the authentic Song

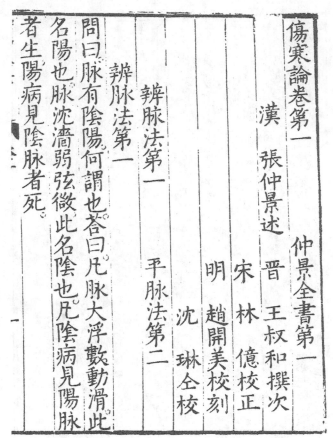

FIGURE 10   Songban Shanghan lun *in the anonymous edition of*
                     Zhongjing quanshu *from the late Ming to early Qing*
                     period. (*Book number 45-13, Cabinet Library, National*
                     Archives of Japan, Tokyo)

style. These two lines and also the line "revised by Lin Yi" (*Lin Yi jiaozheng* 宋
林億校正) were removed from Yang's cut-and-paste edition. Because of these
removals, the number of lines in the edition decreased, and this caused the
center of the woodblock to shift from its original position. To fix this, the original woodblock center was cut out and a new white center with a "fish tail"
(*yuwei* 魚尾) sign was added. For each page, there were five to six cut-out pieces, and these pieces were recombined by being pasted onto paper. The result of
all this was the cut-and-paste edition in the National Library. Since the pieces
were pasted onto Chinese mulberry paper, the actual work of cutting and past-
ing was done in China. It should be obvious to the reader who was responsible
for this work.

The cut-and-paste edition contains Yang's bibliographic remark from 1913. In it, he laments that although he was able to produce a reprint of the document, no one appreciates its value, and therefore, his objective remains unfulfilled. The "reprint" mentioned here must refer to the Wuchang edition published in 1912. By 1913, Yang had evacuated to Shanghai, and from the above remark, it seems that no one was aware of the existence of the Wuchang edition. Due to the hardships of living as a refugee, Yang eventually had to let go of the cut-and-paste edition. He at some point added the bibliographic remark to it and passed it on to Zhang Shiyuan and Zhang Qinpu, whose ownership stamp can still be seen on the document. However, the Zhang family's *Shiyuan zangshu zhi* 適園藏書志 (*Catalog of Shiyuan's Books*), published in 1916, describes the document as a Japanese copy and expresses doubts concerning Yang's claim: "Although Yang says that the document is based on the Northern Song edition, there is no evidence of this."[24]

Perhaps because people doubted its authenticity, no one paid much attention to the Wuchang edition of *Shanghan lun*. However, there were a series of publications of *Shanghan lun* following the Wuchang edition. Yun Tieqiao 惲鐵樵 of Shanghai published a facsimile of what was claimed to be Zhao Kaimei's *Songban Shanghan lun* in 1923, followed by another publication, by Shanghai Zhongyi shuju 上海中醫局書局, in 1931. In 1955 *Xinji Songban Shanghan lun* 新輯宋本傷寒論 (*Newly Published Song Edition of Shanghang lun*) was published by Chongqing renmin chubanshe 重慶人民出版社. Judging from the quality of characters and phrases in these editions, it is evident that their source book is not the actual Zhao Kaimei edition but the Horikawa edition. Whatever the case, the Wuchang edition seems to have played a pivotal role in raising people's interest in Zhao Kaimei's *Songban Shanghan lun* in China.

Conclusion

In this essay I have examined Yang Shoujing's large collection of rare medical books purchased from the Kojima family during his stay in Japan and his publication activities after returning to China, which involved both collation and reprinting of the obtained texts. Yang's goal was to make these books recognized widely in China. I have also pointed out that in order to stress the rarity of his texts, Yang presented Ming and Yuan editions as Song editions and also manipulated some of the texts. Finally, I have analyzed the hitherto-neglected

---

24   Okanishi 1969, 355.

influence exerted on Yang by the Kojima family's scholarship. The following is
a list of Japanese authors to whom Yang refers in his *Fangshu zhi* and the number of times he refers to them:

Naokata / Gakko / Hōso (15)
Kojima (2)
Shunki (Naomasa) (1)
Mori / Tatsuyuki (10)
Taki (3)
Nishiki Kōji 錦小路 (1)
Asada Koretsune 淺田惟常 (1)

As should be clear from this, Yang referenced members of the Kojima family
significantly more often than the others. These references furthermore were
often accompanied by Yang's words of praise for the Kojima scholars. I cite a
few examples:

> *Mingtang jing*—"the handwritten copy of Kojima Naokata is extremely
> precise, allowing the reader to get a feel for the original manuscript and
> the handwriting of the Tang author."
> *Qianjin yifang*—"Naokata wrote his collation notes in the margin of the
> first printed edition from the Medical School using vermilion ink ....
> [T]he work was completed after about twelve years. One does not need to
> be reminded of his precision and accuracy."
> *Maijing*—"Kojima collated this using vermilion and blue ink.... [H]is
> work is precise and intricate."
> *Zhouhou fang* 肘後方 (*Handbook on Prescription*)—"Kojima Naomasa
> put together a supplementary edition of this and revised this work in
> intricate detail."
> *Zhubing yuanhou lun* 諸病源候論 (*Theory on the Cause of Various
> Diseases*)—"Kojima Naokata relied on the Song edition .... [H]e made
> over several thousand revisions. His work represents an epitome of preci-
> sion, and there is no room for criticism."
> *Qianjin baoyao* 千金寶要 (*Precious Recipes Worth a Thousand Gold
> Pieces*)—"Kojima Naokata made many collation notes with vermilion
> ink."
> *Waitai miyao fang*—"Kojima investigated piles of books, overlooking
> nothing."[25]

---

25   Yang (1901) 1967, 587–657.

The Kojima family's work on collating and publishing medical classics had deeply impressed Yang. In comparison, Yang's references to Mori Tatsuyuki, the runner-up in terms of the number of references, are mostly simple citations of Mori's analysis of medical texts. In studying Yang's own work on medical classics after returning to China, we need to consider the influence the Kojima family's scholarship had on him.

But why was Yang so persistent in his work of collating and reprinting medical books? What is helpful here is to recognize that Yang devoted himself to the work that the Edo Medical School left unfinished. The collation and publication of *Daguan*, for example, was of profound historical significance, although it was Ke Fengshi who played the leading role. Yang, having learned of the Edo Medical School's large-scale project of collating and reprinting rare medical books, felt the need to carry on a similar project in his own country.

Reprinting rare books, however, requires financial power. This led Yang to cooperate with Ke in the publication of the Wuchang editions. Ke, who owned a Ming edition of *Jiayi jing* with detailed annotations by Kojima Naokata and Naomasa (now owned by the Chinese Academy of Chinese Medical Sciences 中國中醫科學院藏), also praised the work of the Kojimas as extremely accurate and detailed. Following the Sino-Japanese and Russo-Japanese Wars, Chinese intellectuals began to pay attention to—and began to be wary of—Japan's advancement. Chinese intellectuals were also becoming aware of the need to discard their traditional Sinocentric complacency. Within these larger developments, Yang and Ke recognized the importance of rare classical texts and sought to carry on the work of collation and publication that remained uncompleted in Japan. Their endeavors were also partly motivated by a desire to analyze rare books from Japan side by side with classic texts in China and accomplish more effective collation.

However, time was against them. Ke died immediately after the 1911 revolution. Yang traveled to Beijing seeking a government position in the Republic of China but died shortly thereafter before fulfilling this hope.[26] Their contributions should not be understated, nonetheless. Many books that had lost value in Japan were collected by Yang and subsequently bought by the government of the Republic of China, preventing these books from being lost. As mentioned earlier, the scholarly value of the Wuchang *Daguan* is also immeasurable. Today, these books that Yang and Ke helped preserve are once again serving the needs of scholarly communities in the Chinese cultural sphere (*kanji bunka ken* 漢字文化圈).

---

26   Chen 2001.

References

Chen Jie 陳捷 1997. "Shinkyaku hitsuwa" 清客筆話 [Conversations through writing with a guest from the Qing], in Xie Chengtren 謝承仁 ed., *Yang Shoujing ji* 楊守敬集 [Collection of Yang Shoujing's works], vol. 13. Wuhan: Hubei renmin chubanshe.

———— 2001. "Yō Shukei to Ra Shin'gyoku no kōyū ni tsuite—Yō Shukei to Ra Shin'gyoku ate shokan wo tōshite" 楊守敬と羅振玉の交友について―楊守敬の羅振玉宛書簡を通して [On the association between Yang Shoujing and Luo Zhenyu: Examining letters from Yang Shoujing addressed to Luo Zhenyu], *Shoron* 書論 32: 126–138.

———— 2003. *Meiji zenki Nicchū gakujutsu kōryū no kenkyū* 明治前期日中學術交流の研究 [A study of academic exchanges between Japan and China in the early Meiji period]. Tokyo: Kyūko shoin.

Ishida Hajime 石田肇 1990. "Yō Shukei to Mori Tatsuyuki" 楊守敬と森立之 [Yang Shoujing and Mori Tatsuyuki], *Shoron* 26: 163–173.

Kimura Kouichi 木村康一 and Yoshizaki Masao 吉崎正雄, eds. 1970. *Fukkoku bon Keishi hōrui Taikan honzō* 復刻本經史證類大觀本草 [Reprint of *Classified materia medica of the Daguan period*]. Tokyo: Hirokawa shoten.

Kosoto Hiroshi 小曽戸洋 2004. "Kōshō igaku no hitobito to sono gyōseki" 考證醫學の人々とその業績 [Proponents of Evidential Studies of Medicine and their achievements], *Kyōwu* 杏雨 7: 93–107.

Liu Ousheng 劉禺生 1960. *Ji Yang Shoujing xiansheng* 記楊守敬先生 [In memory of Master Yang Shoujing]. Beijing: Zhonghua shuju.

Machi Senjurō 町泉壽郎 2004. "Igakukan no kiseki" 醫學館の軌跡 [The trajectory of the Edo Medical School], *Kyōwu* 7: 35–92.

Mayanagi Makoto 眞柳誠 2006. "Chō Kaibi no Chūkei zensho to Sōban shōkan ron" 趙開美の『仲景全書』と『宋板傷寒論』 [Zhao Kaimei's *Zhongjing quanshu* and *Songban Shanghan lun*], *Journal of the Japanese Society for the History of Medicine* 52: 144–145.

———— 2008. "Yang Shoujing to Kojima ke: Koiseki no shūshū to kōkan" 楊守敬と小島家:古醫籍の蒐集と校刊 [Yang Shoujing and the Kojima family: Collection and publication of medical classics], *Tōhō gakuhō* 東方学報 83: 157–218.

Mayanagi Makoto and Wang Tiece 王鐵策 1998. "Riben Neige wenku suocang de Zhongguo sanyi gu yiji" 日本内閣文庫所藏的中國散佚古醫籍 [Japan's Cabinet Library's collection of medical classics lost in China], *Chinese Journal of Medical History* 28: 65–71.

Mori Junzaburō 森潤三郎 1985. *Taki shi no jiseki* 多紀氏の事蹟 [Accomplishments of the Taki family]. Kyoto: Shibun kaku shuppan.

Mori Rintarō 森林太郎 1979. *Ōgai senshū* 鷗外選集 [Selected works of Ōgai], vol. 6. Tokyo: Iwanami shoten.

Okanishi Tameto 岡西爲人 1969. *Sōizen iseki kō* 宋以前醫籍考 [An analysis of pre-Song medical books]. Taibei: Guding shuwu.

Wang Zhongmin 王重民 1983. *Zhongguo shanbenshu tiyao* 中國善本書提要 [An overview of rare and quality books in China]. Shanghai: Shanghai guji chubanshe.

Wu Tianren 吳天任 1974. *Yang Xingwu xiansheng nianpu* 楊惺吾先生年譜 [A chronicle of Master Yang Xingwu]. Taibei: Yiwenyin shuguan.

Yakazu Dōmei 矢數道明 1977. *Meiji 110 nen kampō igaku no hensen to shōrai* 明治110年漢方醫學の變遷と將來 [110th year of Meiji: The past developments and future of Chinese medicine]. Tokyo: Shun'yō dō shoten.

Yang Shoujing 楊守敬 (1901) 1972. *Liuzhen pu chubian* 留眞譜初編 [The first edition of *Liuzhen pu*], in *Shumu wubian* 書目五編 [Five bibliographies]. Taibei: Guangwen shuju.

——— (1901) 1967. *Riben fangshu zhi* 日本訪書志 [Bibliography of old books obtained in Japan], in *Shumu congbian* 書目叢編 [A collection of bibliographies]. Taibei: Guangwen shuju.

Zhao Feipeng 趙飛鵬 1991. *Guanhai Tang cangshu yanjiu* 觀海堂藏書研究 [A study of the collection of the Guanhai Hall]. Taibei: Hanmei tushu yuoxian gongsi.

Index

---

*   References to the *Treatise* in the index refer to *Treatise on Cold Damage Disorders* (Zhang
    Zhongjing)

Printed in the United States
By Bookmasters